IMPROVING HEALTHCARE TEAM PERFORMANCE

IMPROVING HEALTHCARE TEAM PERFORMANCE

THE 7 REQUIREMENTS FOR EXCELLENCE IN PATIENT CARE

Leslie Bendaly & Nicole Bendaly

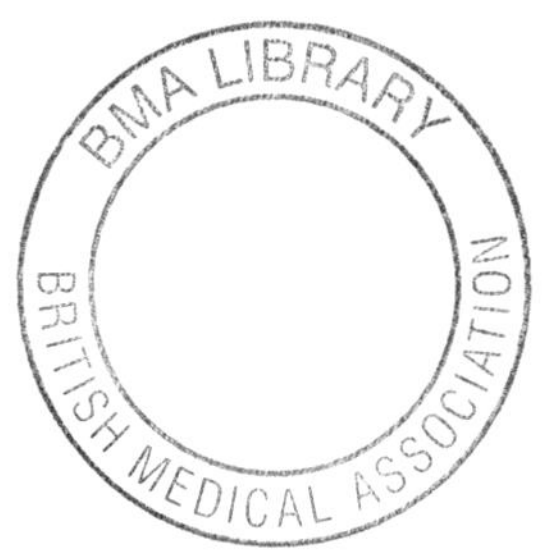

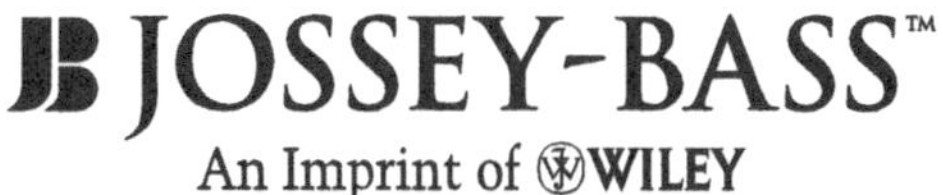

Published by John Wiley & Sons Canada, Ltd.

Library and Canada Cataloguing in Publication Data:

Bendaly, Leslie
Improving healthcare team performance: the 7 requirements for excellence in patient care / Leslie Bendaly and Nicole Bendaly.

Includes index.
Issued also in electronic format.
ISBN 978-1-11819-952-7

1. Hospital care. 2. Patients—Safety measures. 3. Medical errors—Prevention. 4. Health services administration. I. Bendaly, Nicole II. Title.

RA971.B46 2012 362.1068 C2012-902737-5

ISBN 978-1-11819-952-7 (print); ISBN 978-1-11820-972-1 (ebk); ISBN 978-1-11820-965-3 (ebk); ISBN 978-1-11820-967-7 (ebk)

Production Credits
Managing Editor: Alison Maclean
Executive Editor: Don Loney
Production Editor: Pauline Ricablanca
Cover Design: Adrian So
Cover Photography: BananaStock and iStockphoto
Composition: Thomson Digital
Printer: Friesens Corporation

Printed in the United States of America

10 9 8 7 6 5 4 3

To those who work tirelessly to provide quality healthcare and who every day demonstrate their dedication to their patients and colleagues.

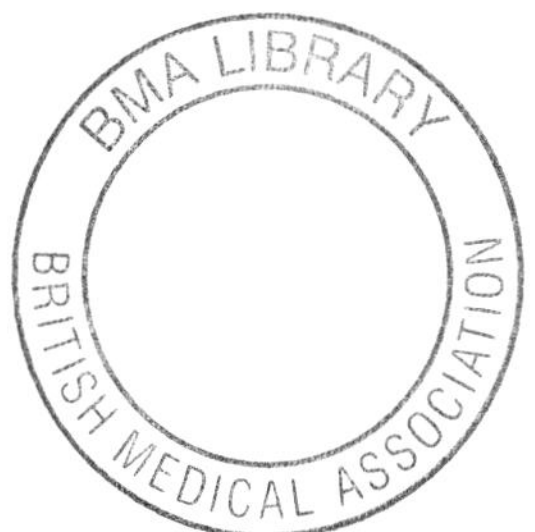

Table of Contents

Acknowledgements

We would like to express our sincere thanks to all who have contributed to this book. We have been fortunate to have met and worked with countless healthcare professionals who have inspired us with their commitment, candour, and desire to help others, and we are grateful to them for sharing their stories so that others can learn from them.

Thank you to Dr. Ken Milne for his passion and dedication to improving patient safety performance and for so generously giving his time and energy to writing our foreword.

We much appreciate Hugh MacLeod, Dr. Ivy Oandasan, Janet Davidson, Dr. Joshua Tepper, Stephanie Leblanc, David Pole, Sandra Ramelli, Michelle DiEmanuele, Patricia Lefebvre and Anne Harvey, who took the time to share their wisdom and experience in transforming healthcare culture so that collaboration and exceptional quality care become firmly woven into its fabric.

The Oncology Program at the Niagara Health System, the New Patient Referral Team at the Juravinski Cancer Centre, Hamilton Health Sciences, and the Toronto Central Community Care Access Centre each participated in the development of this book through focus groups and the sharing of best practices and experiences. What an important contribution they made to our project.

Many individuals contributed to making this a better book. Joanne McNicol provided great feedback on parts of the manuscript, Don Loney, our editor, made valuable suggestions, effectively restrained any verbosity, and polished our prose, and Pauline Ricablanca and her production team did a terrific job of both hunting down our errors and omissions and making the book attractive.

And finally, thank you to Jason and Elie who supported us by sharing the load at home while we focused on the research and writing of this book.

Acknowledgments

Foreword

This book is very timely. Twenty-first century healthcare—with its vastly expanded knowledge base and technologies to manage increasingly complex clinical presentations—has resulted in unprecedented patient expectations. This, coupled with the need to deliver high-quality patient-centred care in a cost-effective manner, cannot be shouldered by one healthcare provider at a time. We have, for some time now, reached the point where the quality of care that patients and families receive depends not only on the knowledge and skills of the individual care providers, but also on the ability of the entire healthcare team to communicate and work well together in order to coordinate the care that the patient/family needs.

Leslie Bendaly and Nicole Bendaly have leveraged their extensive experience and expertise in building effective high-performing functional teams in a variety of organizational structures and applied this to the healthcare environment. They have done this with clarity, mapping out the elements of high-performing teams and showing how each of these elements is independent and yet collectively linked. It is really like an anatomy dissection illustrating the linkage of all the individual parts.

The other important aspect of their book is devoted to providing the strategies, or, as some would call it, a "play book," on the "how to" achieve high performance in healthcare teams. This, in my opinion, has been lacking in healthcare development. Much has been written about what defines a high-performing team and how to measure performance, but little attention has been paid on how to achieve this important construct in healthcare. The solutions the book offers are wide-ranging in scope, from team development processes, balancing behavioural tasks, and process tasks, to the importance of facilitating and nurturing the growth of teams.

The authors also emphasize the importance of leadership in successfully improving healthcare team performance. From my own personal observations and experience, this is fundamental to sustained success of high-performing teams and the impact this has on the provision of safer healthcare. As they so ably demonstrate, leadership in healthcare organizations, as in any other work environment, sets the values and shapes the attitudes that drive the behaviours that in turn drive the performance. Positive behaviours result in high-performing teams, which positively impact patient-care outcomes and cost efficiencies. With negative behaviours the opposite occurs.

Effective leadership walks the talk; leaders behave with integrity and are credible. The credibility is achieved because effective leaders consistently do what they say they are going to do. Great leaders display energy and they energize those around them. As well, great leaders are passionate about mentoring growth.

Leslie and Nicole have captured all of these important attributes of leadership and demonstrated how they are pivotal in building and sustaining high-performing teams. Their work also highlights that it is not just the "C" suite or senior administration team that is responsible for leadership in healthcare—it is, rather, a responsibility that must be shared by many throughout our healthcare structures. In truth, we can all lead from where we are. Leadership is about influence. Leadership is about leading change. If we were all to integrate the behaviours and attitudes that are the component parts of the seven elements required for excellence in healthcare team performance as described in this book, then our progress in providing quality, safe, and cost-effective healthcare would be dramatically expedited.

The book has been written with real narratives from patients and healthcare providers, making it human, relevant, and causing us all to reflect on why we must never give up on trying to improve team performance in healthcare. The use of quotes from notable leaders from many walks of life reinforce the need for all of us to carry and project a positive attitude every day in all aspects of our work. Reading this book will provide direction and guidance for anyone in healthcare, from the front-line workers to senior administration and boards, on how they can raise their participation bar in their own team performance or be more effective in providing leadership for team performance. In doing so, all patients and their families will benefit.

Ken Milne
MD, FRCSC, FSOGC, FACOG

Introduction

This is a book written with purpose and hope. Much has been researched and published about teamwork and collaboration as the essential ingredients in the nurturing of committed, focused, and empowered staff who together provide exceptional patient care. It is theory headed in the right direction. Our purpose in writing this book is to go beyond theory and to provide the knowledge and tools with which one can develop truly collaborative and high-performance healthcare teams, rather than groups that simply carry the "team" name, and to do so with greater ease. Many healthcare leaders have made huge strides in their development of patient-focused teams. Our hope is that the knowledge we share will encourage, perhaps even inspire, leaders and their organizations to embrace teamwork with even greater commitment and vigour.

During our 25 years of working with leaders and their teams, we have found that the importance put on teamwork in healthcare has waxed and waned, sometimes due to the introduction of different approaches to quality care and sometimes due to budgetary constraints.

The intense and consistent focus that has been put on teamwork and interprofessional collaboration in healthcare over the last few years is an encouraging sign that the enormous benefits that are reaped by taking a deliberate and committed approach to developing a team-based culture have been recognized by those dedicated to the profession.

Research shows that nurses who believe that their team is well-functioning have higher levels of job satisfaction, are more likely to stay in their jobs, and demonstrate lower levels of stress and burnout.[1] Another important finding is that higher levels of teamwork have been linked to higher quality care, improved patient outcomes, and an enhanced patient experience.[2] In a study conducted by Donald C. Cole, et al., that investigated the understanding, collection, and use of Quality of Work Life (QWL) indicators in Canadian healthcare organizations, one of the participants articulated the importance of teamwork in maintaining a healthy work environment:

> To provide [the] best patient care, staff need to take into consideration what patient needs are. What does it take to do that?

> There has to be teamwork. There have to be integrated teams. There have to be staff who feel valued. It's all centred around making life better for the patient. If you have a happier group of people, working in teams, you'll have a better end product.[3]

While ideally the development of a team-based culture is an organizational priority, we more often see unit managers and directors taking it upon themselves to improve the effectiveness of their teams. Happily, there is forward movement, but there are still many organizations and leaders who have not made sufficient headway toward creating a team culture. These organizations may be struggling to achieve true teamwork due to any of the following unnecessary blocks that we see every day:

- A misunderstanding of what teamwork is all about (it goes far beyond team dynamics)
- Insufficient endorsement from the senior management of teamwork as a priority (as we will explore, however, this should not stop individual team leaders from taking their groups forward to reap the benefits of true teamwork)
- Lack of team development knowledge and skills
- A false belief, or perhaps hope, that a single intervention or team-building activity can turn a group into a team
- Lack of commitment and follow-through

We strive through this book to provide the know-how to prevent or remove these blocks so that leaders gain the ability to develop and sustain true teamwork within their units and across the organization.

THE 7 ELEMENTS OF A HIGH-PERFORMANCE HEALTHCARE TEAM

Our commitment to team-based culture in healthcare began in the mid-1980s, when Leslie was invited by the Ontario Hospital Association to deliver her intensive five-day program on teamwork to hospitals across the province. This sparked our passion for teamwork, which led us to conduct ongoing research into team effectiveness; to work with hundreds of teams in Canada, the United States, and other countries, both within and without the healthcare sector; to publish several books on the subject; and to develop our now-classic Team Fitness Test, a tool used by teams around the world to measure and improve team performance.

Early on it became evident that teams that were high performing had much more going for them than just good team dynamics. Although a healthy dynamic is essential, other ingredients also need to be present in order for teams to make a powerful contribution to their organization. As demands on healthcare organizations have changed and increased over the years, so have the areas in which teams must excel in order to provide the best patient care.

When the Society of Obstetricians and Gynaecologists of Canada (SOGC) and Salus Global Corporation (Salus) invited us to support their obstetrical patient safety program, MORE^{OB}, by developing instruments to measure culture and communication, we had the opportunity to collect data from hundreds of healthcare workers in Canada and the United States through questionnaires, interviews, and focus groups. The result was data that not only shaped the instruments now being used by Salus to successfully improve patient safety in hospitals across North America, but also reconfirmed the essential nature of what a high-performance healthcare team looks like, including its specific behaviours and practices.

Seven elements are essential to team success and the delivery of exceptional patient care:

- Healthy Climate
- Cohesiveness
- Open Communication
- Change Compatibility
- Team Members' Contribution
- Shared Leadership
- Shared Learning

When a team performs consistently well within each of these elements, both the patient and the team win. When any one or more of these elements are weak, the team experiences challenges that either directly or indirectly impact the patient experience, the quality of patient care, as well as the wellbeing of the team's members. These elements and the tools to help leaders strengthen each make up the heart of this book.

More than healthy team dynamics goes into making an effective patient-focused team.

WHEN TEAMWORK IS LACKING

When we are invited to support the development of a healthcare team, the request is usually triggered by the leader's recognition of some level of dysfunction within the team. The dysfunction most commonly relates to poor team dynamics—ineffective communication, stress-inducing interpersonal relations, and conflict. Although there are critical team requirements in addition to healthy team dynamics, when the dynamics create dysfunction, they become the team's singular pain point.

Although the need for team development is usually identified from internal indicators, the need is actually most urgently evident in the quality of patient care and the issues surrounding it. Is the number of harm events decreasing or increasing? How are mistakes, whether near misses or actual harm events, managed? Are they talked about and learned from in order to prevent them from happening again, or are they hidden due to fears of judgment and blame?

Equally important an indicator is the total patient experience. This may be an even stronger measure of the team's effectiveness, as it is something that is constantly, and too often unconsciously, being created by the team. From an organizational and management perspective, a healthcare organization's reputation for its commitment to quality is a key criterion for individuals choosing a healthcare service provider.[4] And how does the patient define quality? Fred Lee, author of *If Disney Ran Your Hospital*, emphasizes that from the perspective of the patient, quality is not defined by the hospital's patient-safety record "any more than airlines win the loyalty of their customers on the field of who has the best safety record." How they are treated as people and their total care experience are patients' first considerations when defining quality.

From the perspective of the caregiver, who deliberately chose to belong to a caring profession, it is disillusioning and discouraging if their work environment is not conducive to creating a caring experience. From the patient's perspective, it is painful if the one place where they greatly need and expect to receive true care is incapable of offering it.

* * *

Many people have shared their patient experiences with us over the years. Some experiences are positive and illustrate the best of healthcare. Others ask the question, what happened to the *care* in healthcare?

We share the following recent story, written by a patient, because it is a vivid example of a patient experience in which teamwork, collaboration, or compassion for the patient was lacking. While it did not lead to a harm event, it is the kind of example that should be recognized as a critical call for the development of collaboration and teamwork.

6:26 p.m.

A first-time mother is dazed and is starting to feel the beginnings of fear settling in as her midwife works to free her child's neck from the umbilical cord. She anxiously awaits the sound of her son's cry as the midwife passes him off to the physician who works to help him take his first breaths. Finally, after what feels like hours, she hears a soft cry and is temporarily relieved, but then suddenly everyone rushes from the room with her son without so much as a glance in her direction or an explanation as to why. Her husband hurries after the medical staff to the neonatal intensive care unit (NICU), leaving the mother alone in the room. She is in shock but wills herself to have faith that her son will be fine. Her husband returns with pictures of their tiny baby boy in an incubator attached to an IV and numerous tubes, but with little information. The midwife enters the room just as the parents begin to talk about calling their family with the news of the arrival of their son. The midwife says flatly, "I wouldn't be calling anyone just yet," and walks away. What

(continued)

does that mean, they wonder? Is it a more serious condition than they thought? Why isn't anyone giving them any information?

Finally, the midwife returns and informs them that their baby's breathing is laboured, likely due to having inhaled meconium during delivery, and his heart rate is low but that all signs are indicating that he will recover well. They are informed that their baby is now in the care of a physician, which physician the parents do not know, and that the mother will be able to go to the NICU once her epidural wears off.

12:45 a.m.

At long last, a nurse arrives to take the parents to the NICU. The mother holds her beautiful boy for the first time and is relieved to feel his warmth and to see that his heart rate had risen and is now maintaining a healthy rhythm. A nurse stops to look at her son's chart and the mother says, "I'm so relieved he's okay. Will we be taking him home this morning?"

The mother once again feels the beginnings of fear settling in when the nurse, barely looking up from her son's chart, says bluntly, "No, your son won't be going home for a while. He has a boot heart."

"I'm sorry, what did you say?" ask the parents in unison.

The nurse responds in a flat, almost distracted tone: "The X-ray shows his heart is shaped like a boot and he will have to see a neonatal cardiologist and most likely have several more tests."

The first-time parents, who by this point had been awake for over 36 hours, are stunned. Fighting away tears, the mother asks to see the doctor right away and is informed that it is a busy night so she probably won't see the doctor until the morning. The nurse turns and leaves the parents alone holding their sleeping baby with a heart shaped like a boot.

9:30 a.m.

Almost nine excruciating hours later, with still no sleep, the parents see a doctor. The doctor tells them that their son will need more tests, an echocardiogram, and more X-rays that will be sent to the neonatal cardiologist for review. Until they receive the test results, they will not know how serious the condition is or whether it is simply a shadow on the X-ray. The

(*continued*)

parents push for more information: What is a boot heart? How serious is it? What can be done? How common is a shadow on an X-ray? Can't they just take another X-ray right away to double check? They are simply told that there is a range of possibilities and they won't know any details until more tests are done. The physician assures them the tests will be done as soon as possible.

The parents spend the day with their baby in the NICU. No tests are conducted and no physician comes by to check on their son. The nurses are pleasant, encouraging the mother to begin pumping so that she can at least provide her son with important colostrums; however, every time the parents ask to speak with a doctor, they are informed the doctor is busy and will be with them soon. Each time they ask when the tests will be conducted they are given the same answer: "It must be busy up there. I'm sure someone will come down soon to get him."

10:00 p.m.

After a long, anxious day with still no information, the mother goes back to the NICU frustrated and in demand of answers. She spots a woman dressed in pants and a blouse with a stethoscope around her neck. Assuming she is a doctor, the mother asks her if she can look at her son's chart and give her some information about his condition. The physician obliges, and the mother explains that she has been waiting for her son to have tests but she hasn't received an update on his condition. The physician looks at her son's chart and explains that early that morning they received a response from the neonatal cardiologist indicating that it was in fact a shadow on the X-ray and that the child is fine. The physician looks surprised that nobody has informed the mother of the news, and that she and the baby are in fact still in the hospital at all. The physician instructs a nurse to move the baby into the mother's room right away and to discharge them first thing in the morning. The physician walks away.

The mother goes back to her room. Nearly three hours later, a nurse wheels the baby in with not a word to the mother and walks back out. The mother finally allows all of the feelings she has been keeping at bay to wash over her.

(*continued*)

Relief: She can finally take a deep breath having been told that her beautiful boy is healthy.

Trepidation: How do they know for sure that it was a shadow? Had they in fact run additional tests to be sure? Did they conduct another X-ray? What signs should she be looking for that may indicate there may in fact be a problem with his heart?

Anger: Why was it so difficult to get any answers? Why was there so little empathy and compassion shown toward her and her child? What if he did have a heart problem? Would this be the kind of treatment she could expect? Why had it taken so long to inform them that her child was fine?

Frustration: The mother realizes that she had not seen her midwife since the previous day.

Self-doubt: Should she have been more demanding? Should she have pushed harder to get answers? Why hadn't she been more assertive?

Sadness: The first days of her son's life had been made to be far more stressful than necessary. The mother feels that the precious first hours were stolen from her simply due to the fact that nobody took a little time to double-check her son's chart and to keep her informed. Had a nurse double-checked the chart during one of the dozen times she and her husband asked when her son would have his tests, they would have known that the tests were no longer necessary and they would have been discharged early that day. Instead, the nurses made the assumption that "it must be busy up there."

Thankfulness: Her son was healthy and going home.

Gratefulness: The miscommunication did not result in harm to her child.

Imagine this mom's experience had there been collaboration and teamwork in action. Imagine how much more rewarding those shifts would have been to the caregivers had they been working in a team-based environment.

HOW THIS BOOK IS STRUCTURED

In Part I: The 7 Elements of a High-Performance Healthcare Team, we introduce the seven elements required for teamwork and collaboration. At the end of each chapter we provide a checklist to help team leaders and members assess the strength of each element in their teams along with an opportunity for reflection and application of the key learnings from the chapter. In healthcare, where a frenetic pace is the norm, we must actively cultivate the habit of reflection, because without taking the time to reflect, people will run on autopilot, doing, for the most part, exactly what they did yesterday without stopping to examine how well their practices and behaviours are working for them and for the patient.

In Part II: Making It Happen, we describe the team-development process, explain leaders' roles and skill requirements in developing their teams, and provide the tools and techniques necessary to facilitate an effective team-development process.

In Part III: The Tools to Make It Happen, we provide team exercises, which we refer to as *workouts*, to develop fit, patient-focused teams. These activities can be combined to create a complete team-development process, or can stand alone and be used during team meetings, group huddles, or at shift change.

Note: All materials in Part III are available for download from our website, www.healthcareteamperformance.com, along with additional tips and techniques for supporting the development of high-performing teams and the development of improved leadership capabilities. Should you choose, you can also receive ongoing team-development updates and tools.

CREATING CHANGE THAT MAKES A DIFFERENCE

Too often when an initiative to develop teams is undertaken, the resulting change is physical rather than chemical. You may remember that a physical change is one in which one or more of the properties of a substance are altered with no real change in its identity. Water freezing into ice is a physical change. In the end it is still the same old stuff—water—and, indeed, should essential conditions change, the ice reverts to water.

In an attempt to foster team development, for example, members may agree to interact more pleasantly with one another and avoid conflict, but if the underlying issues that cause the conflict are not resolved and the core of the team is not strengthened, the result is physical change. There is no sincere or meaningful change; members are going through the motions. The team may initially look different on the surface, but members will eventually revert to old behaviours.

A chemical change converts a substance into a different kind of matter with different properties and composition. Chemical change requires interaction. It creates something new and releases or absorbs energy in the process. Fireworks are an example of chemical change. The following pages provide the formula for chemical change in which individuals become collaborative and groups become fit, vibrant, patient-focused teams.

PART I

The 7 Elements of a High-Performance Healthcare Team

1

When Groups Become Teams

On rare, remarkable occasions, a bonded, effective team just happens. The right group of people with the right chemistry, skills, and attitudes come together, focused on the same goal, and make exceptional things happen quite naturally. Anyone who has ever been part of that sort of team experience remembers it nostalgically as a highlight of his or her career. A certain amount of euphoria is experienced. There is a team high. This type of team experience, however, like other highs and euphoric occurrences, can usually be sustained for a comparatively short period of time. Spontaneous teamwork is often dependent upon a tenuous mix of elements. As new elements are introduced into the group, or others removed, the cohesion dissipates, and members feel a sense of loss when things change. Group members ask, "What has happened to our team? Why can't we be the way we used to be?" In most groups, the magical mix of elements is not automatically present, and members have to set about actively creating collaboration and teamwork.

Healthy team dynamics are essential to the kind of care that patients deserve and healthcare teams aim for. In the 1940s, Kurt Lewin, who is often cited as the founder of the scientific study of groups, coined the term *group dynamics* and described it as the way groups and individuals act and react to changing circumstances. Since then various definitions of the term have evolved, such as, "Team Dynamics: Often referred to colloquially as 'team chemistry'; the patterns of interaction among team members that determine team spirit, harmony, cohesion, and morale" (*The Oxford Dictionary of Sports Science & Medicine*).[1] We define team dynamics as interactions that influence attitudes, behaviours, and ultimately performance. However, more than dynamics determine a team's performance. The requirements we present in this section include those that affect team dynamics and subsequent and essential collaboration, but also include other factors within the team's control that affect the quality of performance and ultimately the total patient experience.

Frequently what one assumes to be a team is, in fact, not a team, but a group of individuals who happen to be taking up the same space but each going in his or her own direction and working relatively independently of one another with little collaboration. Here's an example: The mother of a young child being cared for by several specialists in the transplant unit was concerned about the extreme pain her child was experiencing. She was told by the pain specialist that the pain was a neurological issue. When asked, the neurologist said it wasn't a neurology issue and that the mother needed to speak with the pain specialist. The lack of collaboration between the specialists left the patient in distress and made the mother a helpless go-between, frustrated by the obvious lack of interprofessional teamwork and collaboration. In this situation the individual professionals may not consider themselves a team as they do not care for patients together on a regular basis; however, if they are to provide exceptional care they nonetheless must collaborate and operate as a team when they do.

WHEN A GROUP BECOMES A TEAM

The degree of "teamness" (as outlined in Figure 1.1) present in a group depends on the degree of commonality of the goal, degree of interdependence of team members, degree of norms and shared meanings, and the effectiveness with which members work together. Effective longer-term or ongoing teams have an advantage in that they have a greater opportunity to develop shared meaning and greater cohesiveness as members learn about and from one another over time.

Groups and interactions are disadvantaged when collaboration does not exist. The resulting outcomes fall below the capability of the members. When there is a lack of collaboration, each member's potential contribution is not realized, and the results can be best described as $2 + 2 = 3$ or less.

On the far right of the continuum, a highly effective team creates synergy. The best of each member is tapped, and experience, knowledge,

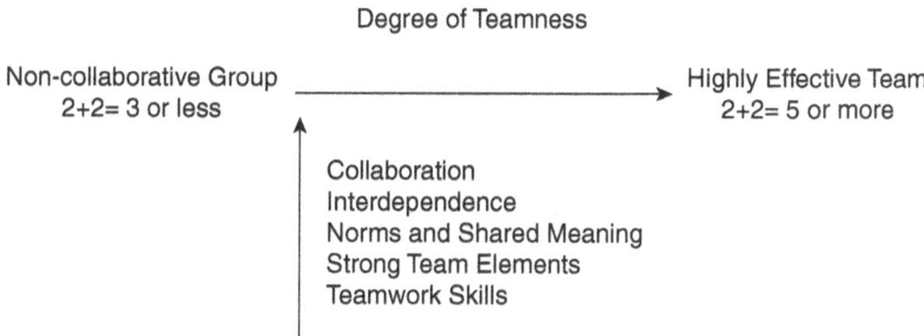

Figure 1.1: Degree of Teamness

learning, and perspectives interact to create much more than the sum of the parts. 2 + 2 = 5 or more. In this case, each of the seven elements essential to high-performance patient-focused care is demonstrated.

> Synergy allows the alliance to be more than the sum of its membership. It accounts for the blending, not just mixing, of the perspectives.
>
> —A.W. Pike

THE ELEMENTS OF HIGH-PERFORMANCE, COLLABORATIVE TEAMWORK

The chapters that follow describe the seven elements vital to high-functioning patient-focused teams:

- Healthy climate
- Cohesiveness
- Open communication
- Change compatibility
- Team members' contribution
- Shared leadership
- Shared learning

Each element is described in Table 1.1. The elements are interdependent; the strength of one can influence the strength of another. For a

Table 1.1 The 7 Elements of a High-Performing Team

Healthy Climate	Healthy Climate refers to how members feel about the way the team functions, including their level of comfort with team norms of behaviour. If the climate is not positive, honesty and openness are lacking and team members may not fully trust and respect one another.
Cohesiveness	Cohesiveness refers to the degree to which the team pulls together in the same direction. Cohesiveness requires agreement and commitment to *what* the team is in place to achieve (mandate, goals, and objectives), as well as *how* it will achieve them (values, priorities, and procedures).
Open Communication	Poor communication within healthcare organizations is cited as a major contributing factor in patient-safety incidents. The degree of open communication is reflected by a team's ability to communicate clearly, accurately, and respectfully, with the freedom to express opinions and to ask questions.
Change Compatibility	The team that thrives today must be able to maintain high performance in an environment of accelerated and constant change. Change compatibility requires receptivity and adaptability to change.
Team Members' Contribution	Team members' contribution is determined by the degree to which team members individually contribute to the team's success by fulfilling their team responsibilities. Examples include keeping one another informed, sharing the load, and actively participating by looking for opportunities to improve the team's ability to provide quality patient care by sharing ideas and concerns.
Shared Leadership	Shared leadership requires that each team member is appropriately self directed, involved in the decision making process and is an equal member of the team in that their input is both valued and respected.
Shared Learning	Learning is at the heart of a culture focused on team performance and patient safety. This element measures the degree to which the team actively reflects on experiences, shares knowledge, and provides feedback in a blame-free, "what can we learn from this" manner, so that learning becomes part of the team's regular day-to-day practice.

team to develop effective communication, for example, it must be allowed to interact in a healthy climate where team members trust and respect one another. At the same time, if communication is open and effective, it is much easier to develop a healthy climate.

Since collaboration is a given in teamwork and requires trust, respect, clear roles, and effective communication, some of the elements vital to effective teams apply specifically to collaboration, and may be useful in developing more effective relationships outside of teams as well as within them. The healthy climate, open communication, and cohesiveness elements include the most important requirements for collaboration.

In the following chapters you will find detailed information about each element, as well as a checklist at the end of each chapter to help you assess the strength of each element in your teams.

In order for teams to fully tap their potential, they require a process that supports them in examining and developing each of the seven elements. This process is provided in Part II: Making It Happen. However, if an ongoing process is not immediately possible, you will find many tips and techniques throughout the book to help create incremental improvement in team performance. Furthermore, Part III: The Tools to Make It Happen provides team-development exercises that you can conduct easily during meetings or informal gatherings.

2

Healthy Climate
A Cornerstone of the Staff and Patient Experience

Consider the following question: "On a scale of one to ten, one being low and ten high, how eager are you to get to work in the morning?"

If most members of a team respond with a high rating, the climate is sure to be warm; the unit feels like home, where team members do not have to keep up their guard. It is a stimulating environment in which one can learn and contribute. It is a place where people want to be.

There is a growing body of research that confirms that a healthy climate leads to higher job satisfaction, a healthier workforce (both physically and mentally), lower turnover, higher patient satisfaction, and improved patient outcomes.[1]

Team climate plays a critical role in the patient experience.

Those who work to improve patient safety recognize climate's critical role. Hugh MacLeod, CEO of the Canadian Patient Safety Institute, explains climate as something that can be quickly felt. He describes two intuitive reactions that he may experience within a nanosecond of standing on the edge of a unit. The first reaction is, "It feels good here." The second reaction might be experienced perhaps just 200 metres away in another unit where the only difference is the colour of the paint. There is a similar layout, similar staffing patterns, the same general kind of patients, the same requisition system, the same IT platform, the same supplies.

And yet MacLeod may have the completely opposite reaction: "It doesn't feel good here." The climate is totally different.

MacLeod acknowledges that this isn't anchored to scientific rigour, but the difference is palpable. The difference between A and B, according to MacLeod, is a positive relationship pattern and teamwork pattern. As soon as one enters the unit, one can immediately sense the climate and the energy that the team exudes, whether it be positive or negative. This means that the patient and his or her family can sense it too.

When there is a healthy climate, trust and respect, the two traits that are most consistently identified by healthcare workers as the most critical to effective teamwork, are felt across the team. In a healthy climate team members trust that if they offer feedback, it will be taken as it was intended: to help or to make things better. When members receive feedback, they trust that it is given with the same positive intent. Individual differences in personality type and style are accepted and respected. No one is expected to fit a mould that is determined by a small power group. If someone has a need, they know they can ask. If the individual approached does not provide the required assistance, they trust it is because the person is unable to help at the time. If someone has a question, they trust they can ask without being perceived as incompetent or interfering. Team members see caring for and supporting one another as an intrinsic part of being a team member, and as something that adds to the fulfillment of the job. A warm, healthy organizational climate both energizes and soothes those who live in it.

A WARM CLIMATE

Team Members' Perspectives

A Physician in Adult Rehabilitation:

"We may be a dysfunctional family at times, but at the end of the day we want the best for each other and trust that everyone is doing the best they can with the resources they have at the time. We argue like most families, but in the end we work through it. I wouldn't continue working in a department where we didn't care for, trust, and respect one another."

(continued)

A Nurse in a Children's Hospital Transplant Unit:
"We practise family-centred care where the patient is the number one priority at all times, so there is no ego, there is no jockeying for position, and no pecking order. We are simply just there for the patient, their family, and for one another. It's hard to describe. I never feel alone because there is such a strong sense of teamwork. I know that when I ask for help I'll get it, I know I can always ask questions, and I know that my opinion is valued."

A cold climate depletes energy and puts people in survival mode, bringing out their most negative behaviours. It creates the worst possible experience. Communication may be uncaring, even cruel; gossip may abound; cliques may thrive; some members, for reasons that are often unclear, may be made to suffer, at times, by being excluded or bullied.

A COLD CLIMATE

Team Members' Perspectives

An Emergency Department Nurse:
"Who you are working with greatly impacts whether you have a good or bad day. It's a shame what this department has become. We used to be a close-knit group, but now it is every person for him/her self."

A Student Nurse:
"It was just awful. We were there to learn, to take the load off of other nurses so that we could learn, and we were treated with such disrespect and often pure disdain. There were times when I wasn't even acknowledged. I would actually approach a nurse who was supposed to mentor me and ask her a question, and she would ignore me and just walk away. It was the worst experience I have ever had. Now, thankfully, I know that not all units are like that."

(continued)

A Seasoned Nurse:
"After each shift I go home feeling defeated because I could not efficiently give the care I want to my patients. I don't work in a supportive environment where people trust and respect one another, and that impacts my ability to ask for help and to trust that others will be there when I need them to be."

An unhealthy climate not only depletes the caregiver, but also hinders the quality of care that committed individuals strive to give.

The Healthy Climate Shapers: trust, respect, communication.

Once a chill sets in, the situation inevitably grows worse unless the team takes responsibility for grappling with it and making a change. Whether a healthy climate is unhealthy or simply not as warm as it could—and should—be, three climate shapers require investigation and development: trust, respect, and communication. Trust and respect are discussed below, and communication is addressed in Chapter 4.

TRUST

In his book *Trust in the Balance*, Robert Shaw describes trust as "The belief that those on whom we depend will meet our expectations of them." A nurse in a labour and delivery unit echoes this: "I demonstrate trust in people if they have consistent behaviour and I know what to expect of them." When people work interdependently to provide a high level of patient care, trust is essential to their performing effectively.

Trust develops most easily among people who have a common experiential base. No group has a completely common base because members each bring their own personal experiences to the group. These experiences include the values they learned growing up, which can differ greatly from one person to the next, even if two people have grown up next door to one another. Although diversity can be a powerful contributor to a team, it limits trust when it is not appreciated and understood.

Diversity, not commonality, is the norm in healthcare populations. Diverse professions have always formed the fabric of healthcare. The strong and differing values and expectations of each profession are inculcated from training onward. These lead to particular ways of doing things, priorities that may strongly differ from those of someone in another profession, and unique communication styles. The potential for miscommunication and misperceptions is therefore greater between professions than within professions, and can easily lead to lack of trust and subsequent conflict.

Overlapping roles, hierarchy, status, and a lack of understanding of other professions add to the complexity of developing trust. In a team that lacks a healthy climate, a physician might, for instance, perceive a nurse's attempt to ask questions about a decision the physician has made as an invasion of his or her scope of practice and control, rather than a desire to learn. In interprofessional teams there can be a kaleidoscope of contrasting working and relating styles, practices, values, and paradigms. The mélange is ripe for engendering mistrust.

In addition, a rich mix of nationalities and races make up the staff in most healthcare facilities. The array of values and expectations that individuals take to work with them every day, combined at times with language differences, can interfere with trust building.

Trusting is easier for some people than others. Team members may be hesitant to trust because of their previous life experiences. Unless these individuals are completely confident that they won't be let down, they refuse to trust. Some may have had issues with colleagues that led them to be cautious and mistrustful. That mistrust may have resulted from an intended unfair action on the part of a colleague, or from a misunderstanding when no harm was intended. Whatever the cause, once trust is lost, it is difficult to rebuild. Trust, that essential ingredient in any relationship, can be the most difficult to develop and the easiest to erode. Much better, then, to maintain it in the first place.

Building and maintaining trust is aided by a common understanding of what trust looks like. Shaw identifies three essential dimensions of trust: results, integrity, and concern for others.[2]

- **Results:** Trust is built when individuals, teams, and organizations consistently demonstrate that they are skilled, competent and can achieve positive results. Trust in an individual requires that we believe they are able to meet their commitments to us and live up to our positive expectations of them. For example, if you expect your manager to respond in a non-judgmental way when you report a near miss, and your manager responds as expected, your trust is strengthened.

- **Integrity:** Trust is built when individuals, teams, and organizations walk the talk by demonstrating consistency between their words and their actions. An organization acting with integrity will ensure that its value and mission statements match the actions of the senior executive team down to the front line. A manager promoting the importance of teamwork will act with integrity and build trust within her team when her actions demonstrate that teamwork is important. For example, she holds team members accountable for disrespectful behaviour.
- **Concern for others:** Trust is built when individuals show concern for the well-being of others by
    - Recognizing the impact of one's actions on others
    - Showing a sincere desire to promote the well-being and success of others
    - Showing confidence in people's abilities
    - Recognizing contributions of others

"Praise is infinitely divisible. Give it away every chance you get and there's always plenty left for you."

— Donald Berwick, founder of the Institute for Healthcare Improvement (IHI)

Trust most readily develops within a team when team members recognize and appreciate the unique skills and contributions each member brings to patient care. In order to better understand how trust is recognized in a healthcare environment, we asked more than 200 healthcare workers, including nurses, physicians, midwives, and administrators, to describe how they know when they are trusted. The most common responses to our question "I know I am trusted when…" included:

- I am not second-guessed. My decisions/assessments aren't questioned.
- There is a willingness to work with me under difficult/stressful situations.

- I am asked for my opinion.
- I am given an important task and/or more responsibility.
- People show confidence in my knowledge base.
- My practices are not undermined (i.e., second examiner repeats practice).

We also asked people to share what an environment based on trust looks like, and the following represent the most common responses to our question "I know I work in a team based on trust when . . . ":

- People feel comfortable asking questions without the fear of being judged.
- We are kept in the loop and informed on a regular basis by management.
- Physicians and nurses communicate openly and respectfully with one another.
- I hand a patient over to someone else and they demonstrate the same values in caring for that patient as I do.
- People proactively ask for help.
- People don't undermine others in front of the patient or peers.

"Few things can help an individual more than to place responsibility on him, and to let him know that you trust him."

— Booker T. Washington

When a group is fortunate enough to have a bond of trust, it is easy to take that trust for granted. Maintenance is required to keep a healthy environment of trust within a team, just as it is required to keep a healthy body or a healthy marriage. Maintenance of a trusting environment requires being aware of disagreements that could lead to conflict, and working through those disagreements before relationships deteriorate. Ideally team members should take on this responsibility themselves, and in a well-developed team they will do so. If the team is not yet at that stage, the leader must be tuned in to members' interactions and address issues before they escalate. These "people issues" may not be regarded as high-priority, and may be ignored in the face of what are perceived to be more pressing issues. However, the little stuff can quickly accumulate and turn a good team into a mediocre group.

Where Trust Building Starts

> The place where leaders should start trust building is not within the team they lead but within themselves.

When trust is lacking, renewed trust does not just happen. We must give trust if we expect to receive it. But trusting requires risk taking and, as Shakespeare would have said, "There's the rub." What is the risk if we bring an error or even a potential error to someone's attention? What is the risk if we admit to not knowing something? What is the risk if we fess up to our own error? What is the risk if we voice disagreement? What is the risk if we share what we are really thinking? What is the risk if we share information? What is the risk if we reach out to someone with whom we have had conflict?

The perceived risks can range from damage to one's pride, being seen as a non-team player, being ostracized from a power group, and being seen as lacking skills, to fear of jeopardizing one's position. When the climate is unhealthy, the risk is not only perceived to be high, but is high because members may look for opportunities to find fault with one another. The danger is that mistrust can develop where it is not justified.

The place where leaders should start trust building is not within the team they lead but within themselves. By trusting others, the leader is both modelling trust and establishing an environment in which others can begin to take the risk to trust. Leaders demonstrate trust by being authentic. They believe in transparency and the sharing of information and knowledge; they share power by sharing decision making or delegating leadership tasks. They consistently act with integrity and are more interested in finding the right solution than being "right" themselves. They are self-aligned: what they say and what they do are congruent. They are generous in acknowledging others' accomplishments. They demonstrate respect and caring. When they are wrong, they acknowledge it.

It sounds like a long list, but it basically combines a few skills in communication and participative leadership with positive interpersonal behaviours. Although the leader cannot take full responsibility for a lack of trust in a team, his or her own behaviour is the most powerful determinant of whether the climate is conducive to trust building.

RESPECT

Respect is a value that is expected to be present within any team. It is essential to one's personal well-being, and it is the cornerstone of a healthy workplace. When respect is lacking individuals feel at best devalued and demotivated, and at worst bullied, abused, and harassed. If team members are shown a lack of respect, they feel discounted.

Discounting people saps their energy and confidence, making it difficult for them to be highly contributing team members. Their ability to care for patients and their own physical and mental health is put at risk. Alarmingly, in one study conducted in Ontario, Canada, fewer than 50 per cent of nurses reported that they received the respect they deserved for contributions to healthcare in their organization.[3] This result was replicated in the *National Survey of the Work and Health of Nurses* (*NSWHN*) by Statistics Canada and the Canadian Institute for Health Information (CIHI) (2006), in which perceived lack of respect was identified as a significant predictor of nurses' mental and physical health.[4]

Teams consistently identify respect as key to their effectiveness and central to developing strong interpersonal relationships. Respect, however, can be an elusive term, often referred to broadly as a common need, but not often broken down into specific behaviours and practices so that all team members fully understand what it means to demonstrate respect in their work environment. When we asked the same group of healthcare workers referred to above what respect looks like, we received very common responses, including, "I know I am respected when…":

- I am asked for my opinion by my peers, members of other professions, and individuals of higher levels of authority.
- I am sought out for my expertise.
- I am listened to (sincerely listened to).

- I am empowered to make decisions.
- I am not demeaned or condescended to in front of patients or colleagues.
- My skill set is acknowledged.
- My scope of practice/skill set is trusted and valued.
- I am spoken to in a professional and courteous manner, in attitude, tone, and body language.
- I am treated as an equal by my peers and those at higher levels of authority.

There was also consensus among respondents that greater trust would exist in the team if each individual took responsibility for consistently demonstrating respect. Respect cannot be dictated through organizational policies alone. The conscious decision to treat another person with respect must be made at the individual level. And so, creating a healthy workplace based on respect is within the power of each and every team member. This is good news. Teams do not need to wait for the organization to undertake a new initiative to promote respectful behaviour; teams can promote this themselves by actively demonstrating positive behaviour and promoting zero tolerance for any behaviours that demonstrate a lack of respect toward co-workers and patients and their families.

The need for individual responsibility, however, does not lessen the importance of organizational policies with consequences for inappropriate behaviour. Zero-tolerance policies, with clear expectations regarding what respectful behaviour looks like and clear consequences that are applied to all within the organization, are important, in particular as they relate to violence and harassment in the workplace.

A workplace violence study conducted in 2002 produced results that raised concern throughout the healthcare industry. Of the 461 nurses consulted, 91 per cent reported experiencing verbal abuse in the month previous to the survey. Although most facilities have since made at least initial inroads in eradicating abusive behaviour, the results are worth noting.

According to the study, the most frequent source of verbal abuse was the physician, followed by patients, patient families, peers, supervisors, and subordinates. Not surprisingly, there was a significant correlation between the degree of abuse and the nurse's intent to leave his or her position. This suggests that higher levels of turnover are incurred in environments in which verbal abuse is present.[5]

In a study that investigated the primary factors affecting newly graduated nursing students, the nurses who were surveyed consistently described intimidating and verbally abusive behaviour directed at them by senior staff physicians. In addition, throughout the duration of the study, none of the nurses addressed the disrespectful behaviour either directly with the physician or with the nursing unit manager.[6] This treatment was accepted as part of the work environment. When disrespectful behaviour is tolerated, the behaviour will continue and the climate will quickly erode.

Gaining Respect

We have emphasized the need to show others respect, but in order to create a healthy climate, it is equally important to behave in a manner that is worthy of the respect of others.

Respected team members tend to share a number of common characteristics. They are skilled in their profession, they show respect for others (demonstrate the behaviours described above), they are trusted by others (demonstrate the behaviours described above under "Trust"), and they are ready to support others.

When a team is dealing with the issue of disrespect, it is not unusual to discover that the root of the problem is a failure to understand another person, or an unwillingness to accept that person's idiosyncrasies.

At one time Aboriginal communities in the American Southwest developed a method to prevent the loss of respect. Their primary value was accepting individuals as they were, which simplified getting to know and understand one another. Each individual at birth was given a shield to represent who he or she was. The animals, plants, and elements on the shields represented individuals' personal characteristics.

A story is told of one tribe that, for hundreds of years, followed the custom of hanging an individual's shield on his or her teepee. It is said that, during this period, there was no conflict or war. There could be no misunderstanding; everyone knew and accepted each other's idiosyncrasies. For example, if someone was of the cougar people, it would be known that when cougar people lose their balance, they can be fierce toward anyone that they feel has wounded them. Or if the individual was of the deer people, it would be known that the individual is not comfortable talking about herself or himself. People responded to others according to their characteristics. There was an effort to respect individuals' uniqueness and to hold realistic expectations of them. Individuals did not expect another person to respond as they themselves would have. This did not mean that people were not expected to grow, but that it was each individual's responsibility to recognize their need.

We cannot always transfer practices from one culture to another; however, very often there are important underlying principles that are universal. The key lessons we can take from the power shields are the benefits of

- Getting to know co-workers better as people
- Accepting individual differences
- Recognizing our personal responsibilities as members of a system
- Adjusting our behaviours, when necessary, for the betterment of the community

---

"An enemy is a person whose story we have not heard."

—Gene Knudsen Hoffman

CONFLICT: THE OUTCOME OF DISAGREEMENT IN A COLD CLIMATE

A cold team climate depletes energy and puts people in survival mode, bringing out their most negative behaviours.

It has become popular in human resources literature to talk about good and bad conflict. For our purposes here we define conflict as "unproductive and unresolved differences that harm or threaten to harm interpersonal relationships." While differences of opinion, if effectively explored and managed, are essential to team success, and can produce very positive outcomes, conflict in teams suggests a battle that has no positive outcome.

Interpersonal Conflict: The Negative By-product of a Cold Climate

The nurse-physician relationship is frequently cited as being "conflict conducive." As the nurse's role continues to evolve, and nurses are given even greater responsibility for decision making, some suggest that opportunities exist for increased conflict between nurses and doctors.[7] Instead, in a healthy climate in which people trust and respect one another, this new way of working presents an opportunity for increased collaboration and responsibility sharing.

Opportunities for conflict abound in healthcare far beyond the nurse-physician relationship. Unclear roles and authority, scarce resources, unequal workloads, differing goals and priorities, and power struggles are common conflict triggers between professions and co-workers.

Dealing with Conflict

There are three common approaches to dealing with conflict. In an unhealthy climate, the choices most often made are two extremes: avoidance or confrontation. Neither produces positive results, and each behaviour then adds to the team's dysfunction.

When there is avoidance, the issue is never constructively addressed. In some cases, if the issue is avoided for long enough, it goes away or seems less important. However, the memory of the conflict, and the distrust that it has augmented, doesn't go away. It festers, and so relationships deteriorate.

Confrontation is intended to result in a winner and a loser. Depending on the style of the participants, there may indeed be a winner and a loser. Once again, although the issue may appear to be resolved, relationships have been damaged and the loser is likely to continue to distrust the winner. Another result of confrontation could be a stalemate: nothing is resolved, nothing is accomplished, and interpersonal relations have been weakened.

The third approach to dealing with conflict is collaboration. In a high-performance team, differences that could lead to conflict are managed collaboratively. The issue is openly discussed, mutual understanding is sought and achieved, and there is no thought of winners or losers. The focus is on what is best for the team and, ultimately, quality care.

In a healthy climate, everyone understands that team members take action and put forward ideas with a positive intent. There is therefore no impetus for a negative response. Ideas and actions do not have to be defended. Trust allows members to replace potentially heated discussion with collaborative dialogue that results in new insights and better understanding of one another. Whatever the conclusion, the openness, understanding, and consensus that take place result in all parties leaving as winners.

"Before you speak, ask yourself: Is it kind, is it necessary, is it true, does it improve on the silence?"

—Shirdi Sai Baba

Once a group is functioning as a high-performance team, team members are able to prevent and manage conflict and have learned how to use differing opinions to get better results. However, until the team is well developed, the effective leader must support the team in addressing conflict issues. The less effective leader will ignore signs of conflict and hope that the issue will somehow resolve itself. (Strategies for heading off conflict, facilitating conflict resolution, and getting the best from differing points of view can be found in Chapter 11: Facilitation: The Skill that Determines the Success of the Process.)

MAKING ASSUMPTIONS: THE NUMBER ONE COLD CLIMATE CULPRIT

When the team climate is not healthy, assumptions abound. Assumptions may indeed be our Achilles heel. They play havoc with relationships of all kinds and they cause us to make bad decisions in all aspects of our lives. They lead to harm events and to poor organizational decisions. The frightening thing is that we are not often aware we are making assumptions.

We assume others' motives or intent based on our own experience or values base, which frequently do not match what we are interpreting. For example, in a meeting with a team of occupational therapists, someone raised the issue of a lack of member participation in team committees and meetings. It became evident that a small group of team members were growing resentful because they believed that they were always the ones to step up and take on the workload. They thought that others weren't willing to put the team's needs over their own. This assumption led to a clear divide between those who felt they were always carrying the load and the rest of the team.

Upon greater clarification and team reflection, it became evident that the lack of participation had little to do with a lack of willingness to take on more responsibility, and everything to do with a series of significant changes that left team members feeling disconnected from the team's vision and from one another. The result of this disconnect was that members failed to understand the purpose of the team's committees and their importance to the advocacy of occupational therapy within the organization. This, coupled with the belief that team meetings were unproductive and a waste of time, led to a significant decline in team member participation, and to the perception that these team members had checked out and were unwilling to take on team responsibilities.

Once the team came together to challenge these assumptions and address the issues impacting team member participation, the team's climate improved and participation (along with team satisfaction) began to increase. Teams that most quickly build a positive climate, and curtail conflict in the process, learn to challenge their assumptions before coming to conclusions.

The only assumption we would encourage is the assumption that the intent of fellow team members is positive.

PERSONAL RESPONSIBILITY AND GROWTH IN BUILDING A HEALTHY CLIMATE

It is the collective attitudes and behaviours of team members that create the climate. Stress can play a role in creating an environment in which people react negatively to situations because it is more challenging for them to manage their personal responses. However, stress is not the only culprit. The catalysts for a cold climate are, for the most part, ego, pride, and insecurity, which may be accentuated at times of stress.

Building a healthy climate requires that individuals take responsibility for responding productively to situations and to one another. The following Cherokee parable about an old man teaching his grandson about life illustrates the power individuals have to affect behavioural change and create a positive culture within their teams and organizations.

"There are two wolves fighting ferociously inside me." he said to the boy. "One wolf is evil. He is anger, envy, sorrow, regret, greed, arrogance, self-pity, guilt, resentment, inferiority, lies, false pride, superiority and ego."

"And who is the other wolf, Grandfather?" asked the boy.

"The other wolf is very different. He is good. He is joy, peace, love, hope, serenity, humility, kindness, and all other good things," answered the grandfather.

"Do I have wolves living inside me?" asked the boy.

"Oh yes. You and every living person," said the grandfather.

The boy looked worried. "Which will win, Grandfather?" he asked.

The old man replied, "The one you feed."[8]

Every individual, team and organization has wolves fighting inside them. Not wolves of good and evil but wolves of success, failure and mediocrity. Individuals and teams feed these wolves with the words they choose, the actions they demonstrate, the decisions they make and every little thing they do every day. These wolves don't get fat on one big meal, such as one big success or one big mistake, they get fat on the little crumbs team members drop every day. These crumbs represent the little things that seem inconsequential at the time or are ignored: a near miss might not be reported, an important question may go unasked, a response to a colleague might be impatient, aggressive or defensive, eyes might roll or gossip passed along. Small actions like these feed the wolf of mediocrity and potentially the wolf of failure.

One may think that the wolf of failure is the most dangerous wolf but in fact it is the wolf of mediocrity that is most lethal and often the most well-fed. When we fail we know we have failed and usually take action to rectify the situation. Mediocrity however sets in over time and is less noticeable and therefore teams are less likely to take significant action to improve their performance. Mediocrity, if left to grow, will inevitably lead to errors, poor quality care and poor staff morale.

Exceptional teams and leaders know that the culture in which they work is a direct reflection of the behaviours and practices demonstrated by all members. These teams actively strive to create a culture of success by keeping a close eye on which wolf they are feeding and make a conscious effort to ensure they are consistently feeding the wolf of success and are starving the wolves of failure and mediocrity.

When teams consistently feed the right wolf the climate will strengthen and one of the most and rewarding outcomes is that not only is the team transformed, but the individuals are transformed as well. This happens when team members embrace the practice of reflection that we encourage throughout this book.

> "It's not what happens to us in life that creates our experience but how we choose to respond to what happens."
>
> —Leslie Bendaly

Each of the seven elements required for high-performance teamwork interact with one another. This means that each of the other six elements has an impact on climate. However, it is the teams that exhibit a strong communication element that are the most likely to have healthy climates. We discuss this more in Chapter 4: Open Communication: At the Heart of Quality Patient Care.

REFLECTION AND APPLICATION

Signs that the Healthy Climate Element Is Strong

Leaders can conduct a quick check of their team's climate with the following assessment. Assign a response of Yes, No, or Sometimes to each of the following questions.

Do team members...	Yes / No / Sometimes
...foster an environment of openness and trust?	
...consistently treat one another with equal respect?	
...challenge assumptions and form opinions based on facts?	
...look for opportunities to recognize teammates and celebrate accomplishments?	
...focus more on how they can contribute rather than on what they aren't getting?	
...look for what's right in others rather than what's wrong?	
...manage conflict effectively?	

The climate element requires strengthening when one or more of the above questions is rated a "Sometimes" or a "No."

Reflection and Application for Leaders

1. Developing Trust

> "Trust men, and they will be true to you; treat them greatly, and they will show themselves great."
>
> —Ralph Waldo Emerson

The climate is strongly influenced by the way in which leaders respond to and interact with those they lead. To what extent do your behaviours reflect Emerson's advice? Consider your daily interactions with staff. Do your

(continued)

behaviours reflect trust? Does the way you treat people consistently send the message that you believe in their capabilities and potential? Do your behaviours reflect Shaw's three essential dimensions of trust: respect, integrity and concern for others?

To further challenge your thinking on this question, you might ask for input from those you lead.

2. Combating Stress by Fuelling Your Team

A team's climate can be put to the test when team members feel overworked, undervalued, demotivated, and very tired physically, mentally, and emotionally. When people operate from this unhealthy state, stress increases and there is a higher tendency for team members to demonstrate unproductive and disrespectful behaviours. People aren't necessarily behaving negatively out of malice or disrespect; however, when people are stressed, they aren't operating with a healthy state of mind. This means they are less likely to make conscious decisions when choosing their responses, and may not take the time to consider the best practices and behaviours for various situations.

As a leader, taking steps to create a healthy work environment is a critical responsibility. You can start by carving out a few minutes every week to energize team members. Energy that carries individuals the farthest is created when they are a part of something special and feel good about themselves and one another. Reflect on the following energy boosters and select three that you will commit to putting into practice on a regular basis to energize your team members and combat stress.

Team members are energized when they

- Are asked for input on issues
- Are given regular feedback on performance
- Receive pats on the back (even little ones)
- Are kept informed about important issues, decisions, or happenings
- Work in a positive climate in which people enjoy one another
- Socialize with colleagues
- Have fun

(*continued*)

- Know their manager/leader cares about their well-being
- Are treated with respect
- Are helped to grow professionally
- Have challenging work to do

Reflection and Application for Everyone

1. Reflect on Relationships

Think of someone with whom you do not feel aligned. You may have frequent differences, even conflict, or perhaps the individual simply irritates you.

Identify the qualities or traits in that individual that create in you a negative emotional flare. Reflect on these and ask yourself why these behaviours create a negative emotional response in you.

Very often when others' behaviours irritate us it is because we have been reminded of a personal trait which we are not proud of. One woman was annoyed by a colleague who frequently talked about her latest purchases. On reflection, the woman realized that the conversations reminded her that she couldn't afford those things because she wasn't managing her own money well. Another was irritated by what she thought was her manager's over-the-top focus on detail. On reflection, she recognized that a lack of attention to detail was her own weakness. Her frustration, which was raised by the manager's detail orientation, was actually frustration with herself.

Considering traits in others that annoy us can help us recognize and commit to our own personal change, or at the very least lessen the level of emotion the other individual is able to trigger.

2. Reflect on Respect

Most people know how to show respect, but may not recognize when they are showing disrespect. Ignoring someone's input or point of view, cutting them off in discussion, putting someone down, gossiping, and communicating with a raised tone of voice and aggressive body language tell the individual that they are not respected.

(continued)

We once overheard a member of a team say of another member, "When they earn my respect, they'll get it." Is there someone you feel this way about? If so, how have you shown them disrespect?

Imagine responding more respectfully to them. What change could your respectful manner bring about? Might their behaviour change? Might your modelling positive behaviour increase your peers' respect for you? Whether or not we show someone respect tells more about ourselves than it does about the other person.

3. Feed the Right Wolf

High performance teams are fanatically focused on feeding the wolf of success by ensuring the behaviours and practices they choose reflect those that are in the best interest of delivering exceptional care and creating a positive staff experience. Reflect on the behaviours you demonstrate daily and identify those that feed the wolf of success, mediocrity and failure. For any that feed the wolf of mediocrity and failure identify what you can do to prevent and or eliminate them.

3

Cohesiveness

Achieving the Common Goal of Exceptional Patient Care

When the *cohesiveness* element is strong, team members make music together. A cohesive group is like an orchestra; each member is working in the same spirit and playing the same symphony, but each is contributing very separately and distinctively. Each member is very clear about the part of the score he or she is playing. Each member is using different skills, tools, and techniques, but at the same time they are all in concert.

Cohesiveness is often thought of as sticking together. Sticking together isn't always easy, especially in a complex, fast-paced, high-pressure environment like healthcare, where a variety of professions come together with unique experiences and perspectives. The trick to sticking together is ensuring the right ingredients are in place to create the glue that will bind team members through the ups and downs they will undoubtedly face. The recipe for team glue includes agreement on where the team is going (its goals and objectives) and how the team will get there (its values and best practices).

When roles are clear and agreed to, and priorities and values shared, it is much easier to trust one another. Cohesiveness, then, has a strong influence on the health of the team's climate. Here are essential ingredients that underpin cohesion:

- A clear and agreed-to common goal that is kept in mind at all times
- Clearly defined roles and responsibilities that are understood and respected by all

- Common values that define the team and how it achieves its goal
- Adhered-to agreements as to how team members work together
- Pride in the team

> Cohesiveness requires agreement on where the team is going (its goals and objectives) and how the team will get there (its values and best practices).

A CLEAR, COMMON GOAL

Teams that don't keep their goal in front of them lose their way. Exceptional teams and organizations are focused—very clearly—on where they want to go. High-performance teams keep their goals at the top of their minds at all times and never lose sight of them. Too often, however, once a goal is set, it is stored somewhere in the back of people's minds as the team puts its collective head down and focuses on the day-to-day tasks, stresses, and issues.

A team has a number of goals, including patient, professional, departmental, and organizational goals, along with short-term and long-term goals.[1] The team's overarching goal, however, is the one most important in building cohesion. This goal will relate to the delivery of patient care and will be closely tied to the hospital's vision and mission.

Healthcare teams have an advantage over many teams in other industries in that the goal of quality care is constant and obvious to team members. Ask each member his or her team's overarching goal, and the responses are likely to be similar and will relate to delivering quality patient care.

However, even if each team member knows and recognizes the goal statement, it does not guarantee common understanding. It might seem that a common understanding of an apparently straightforward goal such as quality patient care could be taken for granted. But different teams may have different interpretations, and individuals within the team may envision the goal differently. Members must have the goal statement in mind and a common picture of how it will be achieved through agreed-upon practices, measures, behaviours, and priorities.

A goal that reads "providing quality patient care" will look different in an emergency room than it will in a neonatal intensive care unit. Quality patient care in an emergency room may in part be defined by wait times and efficient triaging of patients, whereas in a NICU, quality care may include supporting the infant's family, as well as providing timely and compassionate communication and updates on their child's condition.

Within a single team, team members may assume they are working toward the same goal, but in practice may have differing and potentially conflicting interpretations of the goal. "Quality" for some may include taking the time to involve the patient's family in decision making, while others may view this as an activity that prevents them from devoting sufficient time to the patient. Their behaviours at times will be quite different, and may lead to conflict and contribute to a lack of cohesion that will hinder team effectiveness.

High performance teams keep their goals at the top of mind at all times and never lose sight of them.

EMBRACING THE GOAL

Janet Davidson, a Canadian leader in hospital administration, emphasizes the need for the quality goal to be understood in practice: "If you have a quality measure, how does that translate to the day-to-day actions of the nurse on the front line?" Davidson also passionately believes that "quality has to be everybody's business and a part of the living, breathing culture of the organization; everybody has to own it."

She explains that barriers to improving quality are created when "healthcare facilities put quality in a basket by relegating the responsibility to the quality department. When 'quality' is somebody else's responsibility, when it isn't everybody's business, people don't take ownership of it. Instead the response is, 'Well, it's the quality department that does that.'" She qualifies that having team members simply buy into the need for quality isn't enough. There must be active involvement in understanding and creating quality.[2]

Defining the Goal

Team members will have a clearer understanding of what is expected of them once they know what the goal is and how it will be attained. They can achieve this understanding by drawing up their own picture of the goal, as well as the behaviours, practices, and measures that are required to achieve it. Once this is accomplished, their commitment to the goal will be greatly increased, and the team will develop a sense of purpose and identity.

The Institute of Medicine has taken steps to add clarity to the definition of "quality of healthcare" by identifying six practices they deem essential to quality patient care. These include care that is safe, effective, patient centred, timely, efficient, and equitable.[3] A team, depending on profession, role, experience, and values, may have a different take on what dimensions best describe quality in healthcare, but the six identified by the Institute of Medicine could be used as a starting point for developing a description of its own goal.

Even if each team member knows and recognizes the goal statement, it does not guarantee common understanding... Highly effective teams use the quality goal as a rudder to steer them to the best choices minute by minute.

Fanatically Focused on Quality: The Quality Goal in Action

Imagine hundreds of clinicians in a facility stopping at the same time to focus on quality.

In 2012 the Canadian Institute for Health Information released the results of their quality-improvement initiative, The Canadian Hospital Reporting Project, in which 21 clinical indicators were used to measure performance and quality. Credit Valley Hospital (CVH), located in Ontario, Canada, scored above the national average in 17 of the 21 clinical

Table 3.1: The Six Dimensions of Quality Healthcare (as defined by the Institute of Medicine)[4]

Safe	Avoid injuring patients with the care that is intended to help them.
Effective	Provide services based on scientific knowledge to all who could benefit from them, and refrain from providing services to those not likely to benefit (avoid underuse and overuse, respectively).
Patient Centred	Provide care that is respectful of, and responsive to, individual patient preferences, needs, and values, and ensure that patient values guide all clinical decisions.
Timely	Reduce waits and potentially harmful delays for both those who receive and those who give care.
Efficient	Avoiding waste, including waste of equipment, supplies, ideas, and energy.
Equitable	Provide care that does not vary in quality as a result of personal characteristics.

indicators, and had the lowest readmission rate in the province. President and CEO Michelle DiEmanuele credits the hospital's consistent and "hard-wired" focus on quality for their results.

At CVH, between 9:00 a.m. and 9:15 a.m. every day, teams across the facility, from executive teams to teams on the units, huddle to check their quality dashboards, each of which has six to eight quality measures. The executive team's dashboard includes measures such as wait time, health and safety of employees, and surgical cancellation. Hand hygiene and infection outbreak are two of the standard measures that sit on the dashboard of each unit. Unit dashboards also include unit-specific measures that are identified by unit team members. In describing their process to us DiEmanuele emphasized that a key success factor is "being so disciplined that from the outside we look boring."

Leaders at CVH ensure there is no opportunity for the quality goal to slip to the back of people's minds. When team members huddle every day to focus together on their common purpose, it not only improves quality, but also works very well to build cohesiveness. This in turn supports enhanced quality of patient care.

Highly effective teams use the quality goal as a rudder to steer them to the best choices minute by minute. Whether the choices relate to a protocol or a team development plan, the question is always the same: *Does this decision (or action or choice) lead to superior patient care (meeting our quality goal)?*

CLEAR AND RESPECTED ROLES AND RESPONSIBILITIES

The hallmark of a true professional is the willingness to leverage the variety of skill sets from multiple professions that are available to a patient.

When roles are not clear, teamwork cannot happen. It takes understanding and respect of one another's roles, appreciation for how they complement one another, and willingness to leverage one another's strengths to function effectively as an interprofessional team. The ability to clearly describe one's own professional role to patients, families and other professionals and to understand the roles of others are such a critical components of effective teamwork that they have been identified as a core competencies for interprofessional collaborative practice by a number of bodies, including the American Interprofessional Health Collaborative, the Canadian Interprofessional Health Collaborative, and the World Health Organization. Other competencies relating to the importance of understanding and leveraging roles and responsibilities include the ability to "recognize one's limitations in skills, knowledge, and abilities," and to "use the full scope of knowledge, skills, and abilities of available health professionals and healthcare workers to provide care that is safe, timely, efficient, effective, and equitable."

When these competencies are not in place, conflicting roles will pose a significant risk to patient safety, quality of care, and teamwork, and can result in increased stress, reduced job satisfaction,[5] and higher levels of turnover among employees.[6] This rise in role conflict comes with the development of interprofessional teams. Sources of role conflict include role ambiguity, overlapping competencies and responsibilities, preconceptions that professionals have of their own role, and stereotyping and misperceptions that individuals hold of members of other professions and disciplines.[7] To a great extent, the success of a team and the quality of patient care is reliant on the diversity of expertise available and applied for the good of the patient. The diversity in skill sets, knowledge, and expertise will, however, go untapped in environments where individuals lack full appreciation and understanding of others' roles.

> "...teamwork requires a shared acknowledgement of each participating member's roles and abilities. Without this acknowledgement, adverse outcomes may arise from a series of seemingly trivial errors that effective teamwork could have prevented."
>
> —Interprofessional Education Collaborative Expert Panel (2011)

Much emphasis has traditionally been put on positions and titles in healthcare, with the result that many in the profession take much of their personal identity and pride from their role. When one's role is not clear, or it is perceived that someone else is trespassing on one's professional territory, it is a potentially threatening situation.

However, when people respect each other's abilities, the patient benefits. Take, for example, a family medical practice that identified the need to reduce wait times for its patients while at the same time providing them with more focused attention. One of the practice's solutions to reduce wait times when the physician is behind schedule was to create the flexibility for nurses to initiate the patient exam when it falls within their scope of practice. If the patient requires a Pap smear, for example (a procedure that falls within the scope of practice of both the nurse and physician), the nurse would have the flexibility to start the exam, thereby reducing the patient's wait time and helping the physician to get back on schedule. Everybody wins, especially the patient. This level of effective teamwork and sharing of responsibilities happens when the following elements are in place:

- The roles and capabilities are understood
- There is specific agreement as to when the nurse can step in
- There is trust between both parties: the physician trusts that the nurse will fulfill his or her responsibilities competently, and the nurse trusts that the physician will support him or her in taking the initiative

When role conflict exists within the team, there is a greater risk of power struggles, turf wars, and confusion relating to autonomy, authority, and decision making—all of which lead to the development of an environment conducive to higher levels of errors and a breakdown in communication and teamwork. When role conflict is present, cohesiveness is absent.

When team members develop a greater understanding of and respect for others' professional roles and responsibilities, it allows them to draw on the expertise of those in other professions, and to share patient-care decisions.[8] They are able to work as a team rather than a group characterized by silos.

A starting point in developing better understanding and appreciation of different roles is to create opportunities for individuals to learn about each other's professions, scope of knowledge, unique functions, and care philosophies. In addition to strengthening cohesiveness, an understanding and appreciation of roles leads to the development of relationships in which each member trusts the knowledge, skills, decision-making capacity, and approaches to care that others bring to the team.[9] As a result, this understanding also strengthens the climate element.

LIVING COMMON VALUES

> Whether or not the team or anyone else knows who they are depends upon the consistency with which they demonstrate their values.

Respect. Compassion. Open Communication. Collaboration. Understanding. Excellence. These and many other inspirational words are used in healthcare facilities every day. They are included in performance management reviews, in mission statements, and in lists of organizational values with the good intention of demonstrating true commitment to a culture in which people work together cohesively to deliver the best patient care possible.

These value-laden words are often seen, if not openly described, as *soft.* Soft stuff seldom gets sufficient attention. The hard stuff that faces us every day gets first priority. The reality is that values are not soft; that is a dangerous misconception. Values are the hard stuff that is required to build a strong foundation. Without them, the structure, whether that of a team or facility, will start to form dangerous cracks.

When you look around the hallways of your facility, do consistently demonstrated values make up the fabric of your team's daily interactions and experiences? Do they embody "how we do things around here"? Often the behaviours that should reflect these values are not given the attention they deserve. When values are consistently translated into action, they greatly increase the team's cohesion.

There is no such thing as a void. If positive values are not actively present, the space will be filled with negative values.

Don't rock the boat. Keep your opinion to yourself. Asking questions is a sign of weakness. A little gossip is harmless. Don't trust management. These sayings won't be found on hospital websites, but these and similar statements are not uncommon on the floor and in the halls of healthcare facilities. They suggest certain rules of engagement that some members live by, and they do reflect values and beliefs, but they are nonproductive ones. These drain rather than energize, and lead to sloppiness rather than meticulous care for both patients and colleagues. When some individuals on a team strive to demonstrate productive values while others demonstrate nonproductive values, the cohesiveness that allows people to pull together cannot exist. When some members don't fully demonstrate support for the team's core values, cohesiveness breaks down and conflict frequently results.

A long-term care team, suffering from interpersonal conflicts and low morale, found that values were a main cause of their dysfunction. The group had come together in an effort to increase its effectiveness. It was made up of several nurses as well as two physiotherapists who spent some of their time on the long-term care unit, and the rest of their time on other units. One issue examined in the team development process was that of work values and beliefs. Since this was a long-term care unit, patients were not there to be quickly cured. Consequently, the team's basic belief was in "the quality of life." They believed in the importance of spending time with each patient, giving each one individual attention, and making each moment as rich and enjoyable as possible.

Most team members contributed enthusiastically to the discussion of their values and how the team could better demonstrate them. One therapist, however, who had been quite participative in other discussions, became quiet. She gradually edged her chair back from the group and soon was sitting almost outside the group as an observer. Her discomfort was obvious. When we probed for her reaction to the discussion, she displayed a good deal of courage. "I realize," she said, "that our values and their inconsistent demonstration are the major source of our problems, and my attitude toward them has contributed to the problem. I intellectually accept the value of quality of life and giving each patient caring and individual attention, but I have difficulty demonstrating it. I became a physiotherapist to make people better. Here, that is not going to happen. As a result, I spend as little time as possible with each patient so that I can get somewhere else where the values are closer to my own. I know others resent this and that my behaviour contributes to lack of cohesiveness and conflict within the group."

In addition to conflict, the team had been suffering an identity crisis. High-performance organizations and teams are clear about *who* they are as well as *what* they do. Who they are is determined by *how* they do things. Values prescribe the *how*, and when they are consistently demonstrated, a team identity is created. Many healthcare teams perform similar tasks. What makes one team unique from another is *how* it approaches its tasks.

This applies on a larger scale to the healthcare organization. The Mayo Clinic, for example, has gained a worldwide reputation for delivering patient-centric care through collaborative multi-professional practice. The clinic gained this reputation in great part due to its ability to foster a culture that promotes the well-being of the patient above all else. Looking back at the history of the clinic, it is evident that the founder, Dr. William Mayo, was a visionary leader well ahead of his time, for in the early 1900s he identified three factors as critical to the clinic's success. These were

- Continuing pursuit of the ideal of service and not profit
- Continuing primary and sincere concern for the care and welfare of each individual patient
- Continuing interest by every member of the staff in the professional progress of every other member[10]

Clearly Dr. Mayo recognized that the clinic's ability to provide the best possible care hinged on being focused on a few critical values.

For many years healthcare facilities have put in place inspirational mission statements and corresponding values. But, too often, like the team's goal, they are not used. They may be proudly displayed on a website or in an annual report, but to spark a cohesive team or organization, they must be used as the torch that guides every member through every day, every hour, and every minute of their practice. In the book *Management Lessons from Mayo Clinic*, authors Leonard Berry and Kent Seltman describe the primary value of the clinic: "The needs of the patient come first." They explain that this value is woven into the very fabric of the Mayo Clinic by ensuring that every decision, every procedure, every process, from the design of clinical and public space to the development and implementation of operational strategies, revolve around that core value. According to Berry and Seltman, this primary value defines the organization's "reason for being."

There is no such thing as a void. If positive values and beliefs that drive teams forward are not actively present, the space will be filled with negative values that will stymie, disrupt, and create dangerous cracks in the foundation of the team. The cracks may emerge as conflict, miscommunication, and low staff morale, all of which can potentially lead to errors. Inevitably, the result is a team that is incapable of consistently providing quality patient care.

The only way to prevent these detrimental values and beliefs—and their resulting negative behaviours—is to ensure the team is chock full of consistently demonstrated positive ones.

DEVELOPING VALUES AGREEMENTS

Bringing team members together to participate in a dialogue about team values and reaching an agreement on which values are essential to team success and the specific behaviours and practices that demonstrate the values is an essential and powerful step in developing cohesiveness. Values agreements define the behaviours and practices essential to living each value so that each team member understands what is expected of them and their teammates.

Getting team members to agree on values is usually quite easy, since values are often expressed as platitudes. Most members of a healthcare team, for instance, would have difficulty saying "I don't agree with improving the quality of life of our patients." Yet each individual might demonstrate the value quite differently, and contribute to the quality of life of the patients to varying degrees.

> Values agreements define the behaviours and practices essential to living each of the team's values.

Just as different values can create conflict, so can agreed-to values that are not consistently demonstrated by all team members. Take, for example, a management team whose members were not working together effectively. The team members came together to re-examine their team values, and they realized that members' demonstration of certain values was the source of much of their dysfunction. They had previously agreed that empowering others was an important leadership value, and they agreed to live the value through better sharing of decision making. Some managers had made a consistent attempt to share decision making, but others had quickly slipped back into their more comfortable traditional style, and continued to make decisions on their own, or, on occasion, involved some colleagues but overlooked other important contributors. Those managers who had taken the time and effort to be effectively participative were frustrated that not everyone was exhibiting their level of commitment. These individuals had difficulty supporting decisions that hadn't been made in a participative way, and thus put these decisions at the bottom of their priority list. This created greater conflict, because the managers who had made the decisions felt that they were not being supported, but did not understand why. As a result, group cohesion broke down.

What had been missing from the discussion of participation as an important leadership value was an honest examination of the challenges that living this value would present. Had they explored these challenges, they might have identified that many managers hadn't had an opportunity to attend learning sessions on how to effectively involve people in decision making. Perhaps they would have considered that these managers might find it easier to slip back into old habits, rather than take on new ones, and would have found ways of supporting one another going forward.

The teamwork values that are most frequently identified by healthcare teams include commitment, supporting one another, equal respect for each member of the team, honesty, and learning together. But no matter what the team values are, they must come from the heart of the team if they are going to be instrumental in its effectiveness, and they must be fully understood and defined by visible behaviours. For example, learning together may be defined by the following set of behaviours: In order to learn together we agree to ask questions, respond to questions in a positive manner, provide feedback to one another, and be open to receiving feedback.

The team has to believe the values are critically important to fulfilling its goal, and not simply words chosen from a list. The values must be agreed to and then demonstrated consistently.

PRIDE

Pride is both an outcome of a high-performance team and a strong contributor to cohesiveness. What people often take greatest pride in is *how* their team and organization do what they do and *what* they believe in. The stronger the team, the greater its pride. The greater its pride, the stronger the team.

Psychologists Timothy Butler and James Waldroop have conducted research showing that many talented professionals leave their organizations because senior managers don't understand the psychology of work satisfaction. They assume that people who excel at their work are happy doing their jobs. People experience ultimate job satisfaction when the job matches their "emotional driven passion" or what the two psychologists have coined "embedded life interests." These do not necessarily determine what people are good at, but they determine the kinds of activities that make people happy.[11]

People whose work is making them happy take pride in what they do, generally excel at it and come to work with enthusiasm that energizes not only themselves but also those they work with and care for.

Ensuring that people are fulfilled in their jobs takes a conscious effort on the part of the leader to get to know each of the people on the team. This requires finding out what motivates them, what makes them happy, and what they would like to see improved or changed.

Leaders who most successfully inspire their people and develope great team pride do so by weaving the team's mission, vision, and values into everyday conversations, and take every opportunity to remind team members of their purpose and of the exceptional work they are doing toward achieving that purpose. Leaders who develop exceptional teams are clear and passionate about their vision and the values that will get the team there, distil them into bite-size pieces, and communicate them incessantly.

A note of caution: once a team reaches a level of high performance, it is not uncommon for team members to begin to take their accomplishments for granted, rather than continue to savour and enjoy them. The energy created by pride and the contribution pride makes to cohesiveness are weakened. Pride is kept alive by sharing success stories, recognizing one another's accomplishments, and celebrating excellence.

Cohesiveness requires the team to agree on the important things that determine how well the team works together and that provide its direction and energy. In Chapter 9: The Team Development Process, we provide a method for developing team agreements that are important to team cohesion. This method can be used for strengthening each of the elements.

REFLECTION AND APPLICATION

Signs That the Cohesiveness Element Is Strong

Leaders can conduct a quick check of their team's cohesiveness with the following assessment. Assign a response of Yes, No, or Sometimes to each of the following questions.

Do team members...	Yes / No / Sometimes
...have a clear and common goal?	
...live common goals?	
...live common values?	
...have clear and agreed-upon roles and responsibilities?	
...demonstrate respect for one another's roles?	
...communicate roles and responsibilities clearly to patients, families, and other professionals?	
...use unique and complementary abilities of all members of the team to optimize patient care?	
...have agreed-upon team processes that guide the team?	
...show pride in being a member of the team/ facility?	

The cohesiveness element requires strengthening when one or more of the above questions is rated a "Sometimes" or a "No."

Reflection and Application for Leaders

1. Get Fanatically Focused on Quality

In order to be fanatically focused on leading your team toward success and consistently delivering exceptional patient care, it is important to know what success means for your team. High-performing teams and leaders are able to state what success is in one sentence. If you can't

(*continued*)

describe it succinctly, you can be sure that those who report to you won't know what it is and will not be pulling together in the same direction to achieve it.

a. Write a success statement for your team and be as succinct and clear as possible. This statement will define the specific objective(s) your team is aiming for.
b. Reflect on and list the values you believe are the most essential to your team's ability to effectively achieve the above success statement.
c. Given your team's success statement and corresponding values, describe how your team might change or improve to consistently demonstrate the values and achieve the team's objective(s).

2. Clarify Priorities

Once you have a picture of success, the next step is to ensure that you have a clear idea of the priorities that you'll need to focus on in order to realize that success. You must know your top three priorities without having to think about them, and your team must also have them at the top of their minds at all times.

Being obsessed with the key requirements for success ensures that you and your team do not get caught up in activities that do not contribute to results. It ensures that everyone is pulling in the same direction.

Having a strong and clear strategic focus provides another great advantage that is not fully appreciated by many leaders. A clear focus increases team members' self-direction, which means members will be better equipped to make decisions on their own. You can then achieve better results faster, with the additional advantage that members will have a sense of ownership (a factor discussed in Chapter 7: Shared Leadership: The Path to Empowered Team Members).

Refer back to your team's success statement and list your team's top three priorities for achieving it.

(continued)

Reflection and Application for Everyone

1. Repairing Broken Windows

Broken windows is a theory in criminology that suggests that if you let little things go they become bigger ones. When windows are broken, vandals are likely to break more. The theory is based on the observation that the existence of broken windows in a neighborhood frequently is found in association with other signs of general social fragmentation and disorder, such as property neglect, disrepair, abandoned cars, overgrown yards, street debris, uncollected litter, and graffiti. In the absence of a sense of community order and control regarding such signs or signals, there appears to be a tendency on the part of local residents to increasingly ignore or even tolerate lesser criminal acts, such as delinquency, drug use, and petty crime.

What broken windows might there be in your team? Any behaviours or attitudes that are not appropriate and go against the team's goals and values are broken windows. They are negative behaviours or attitudes that are being ignored. Perhaps the leader and team members feel they are "little" things compared to other priorities or they hope that they will eventually go away if ignored. A broken window in one team might be disrespectful behaviour, in another failure to follow through on commitments. Organizational broken windows take on many shapes but ignoring them leads to the same outcome. A broken window when ignored sets a low standard of behaviour which discourages committed team members and encourages all to behave as they choose rather than as would be best for the team and the patient. A couple of broken windows can be the beginning of a downhill slide.

1. Make a list of any broken windows that your team needs to repair.
2. Identify how you might contribute to repairing these windows.
3. Share your list of the broken windows at your next team meeting for the purpose of coming to agreement as a team on how to repair them.

(continued)

2. Connecting with Team Members

Reflect on the various professions working within your team, and the variety of skills and expertise available to you and your patients. To generate a better understanding and respect for others' roles, identify individuals and/or professions that you could connect with more regularly for the benefit of you and your patients. Complete Figure 3.1 by placing your name/profession in the centre circle and by filling in the surrounding circles with the names/professions of those with whom you should connect more frequently.

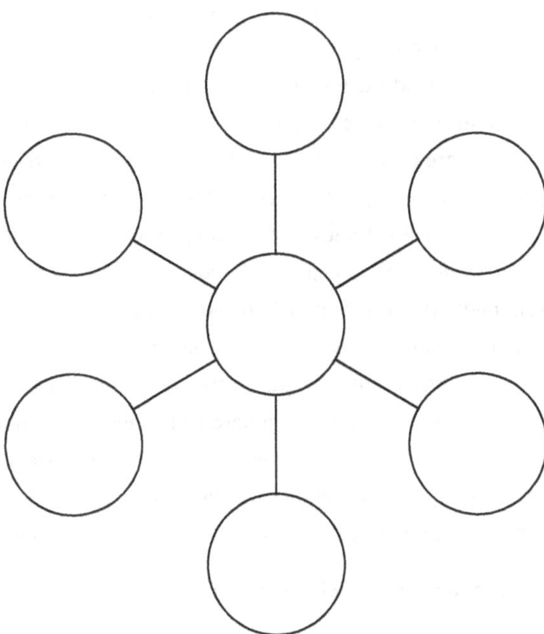

Figure 3.1: Making Connections

4

Open Communication
The Heart of Quality Patient Care

Open communication is essential to any high-performance healthcare team. However, it isn't something that comes easily. Strange, isn't it, that one of the first things we humans learn to do, we often don't do very well at all. Communication can be our greatest strength or our Achilles heel. As individuals, our ability to communicate is the main determinant of our effectiveness and our personal well-being. As part of a team, when our quality of communication is poor the team's ability to perform at its best is significantly compromised. Conflict, frustration, stress, and errors increase; trust, support for one another, and team performance decrease. Good communication in healthcare or any other type of organization seldom "just happens"; it requires conscious effort. Poor communication, on the other hand, usually "just happens."

Research literature has for years identified poor communication as a key cause of hospitals' most serious challenges, which include patient-safety incidents, poor quality care, patient complaints, poor employee morale, and turnover. The Joint Commission Sentinel Database suggests that communication has been identified as a contributing factor in 70 per cent of sentinel events. This is a much higher percentage than other commonly identified factors such as quality of patient assessments or protocol compliance.[1] In a survey we conducted with over 150 healthcare workers, 83 per cent believed that poor communication on their unit affected the quality of patient care over 50 per cent of the time.

There is plenty of incentive to make managing communication processes a priority. However, in today's complex healthcare environment, where patient management involves the coordination of care by a myriad of specialists, and patients may pass through multiple handoffs, it is no wonder that communication breaks down. The challenge of ensuring effective communication is compounded by a multitude of other factors including hierarchy, a lack of role clarity, workload, the organization's culture, interpersonal conflict, power struggles, status, and organizational and professional silos. Many facilities have put processes in place to develop better communication, and other healthcare organizations have worked to ensure that the importance of communication is not overlooked.

In 2005, the American Association of Critical Care Nurses developed standards for achieving and maintaining healthy work environments. The first standard states that "nurses must be as proficient in communication skills as they are in clinical skills."

But communication is a slippery thing and not something easily managed. To manage it well takes an understanding of the impediments to communication, the skills and tools required for effective communication, and a commitment to their implementation. In our practice we have identified six factors that most frequently and powerfully impede effective communication in hospitals:

1. An intimidating hierarchy can prevent people from speaking up. Organizations and professions with long histories struggle more with the issue of hierarchy than do young start-up organizations. Like other organizations with deep roots, hospitals emerged at a time of strict hierarchy throughout society. Classes were distinctly defined, and it was demanded that deference be given to anyone in a position seen as higher than that of oneself, no matter their behaviour.

   The recognition that hierarchy can stifle input, creativity, and, ultimately, performance has led most organizations to acknowledge the need for an open culture in which input can be given freely and in which everyone feels that their contribution is recognized and appreciated. The deeper the cultural roots, the tougher the change process, and few organizations and professions have pasts that go back as far—or as proudly—as those of healthcare.

Although the most cited examples of hierarchy impeding communication, and even leading to error, are interactions between nurses and physicians, any hierarchical situation can limit communication. One study, focussing on resident physicians, looked into how communication errors lead to medical mishaps. The study found that residents' concern about offending those in power (the attending physician), combined with the perception that those with power would not listen to them or hear their point of view, prevented them from productively disagreeing when they had a different point of view.[2]

The issue of hierarchy and communication can be found in any interaction in which one individual is seen as holding a higher status or more power. Hierarchy on its own is not the cause of muddied, incomplete, or lack of communication. Whether or not hierarchy is a communication impediment depends on how the individual in the more junior role views the person in power, and very much on the relationship tone set by the more powerful person. This ties in closely with our second potential communication block.

2. A profession's culture—which begins to be inculcated during training, and has historically been nurtured in professional silos—leads to differing assumptions that can create unproductive communication.

   These may be assumptions about one's own role and assumptions about the roles of others that shape expectations of others' behaviours and their response to oneself. There are also often engendered communication styles. The changes required to shift these culturally based assumptions and expectations take time, and will develop their own roots as new approaches to learning, such as interprofessional education, continue to emerge. In the meantime, great and immediate strides to develop more effective communication across professions can be made from within the hospital, but doing so requires commitment from administrators, as well as from teams and individuals across the facility.
3. When a patient is transferred, the details of the patient's case can be incomplete or inaccurate. This occurs if a patient is handed off hurriedly, or handed off with the false assumption that the individual taking over the patient knows all the necessary information about the case.

Hand-offs have been recognized as dangerous weak spots in patient care, and so have received attention in most hospitals. However, they still warrant vigilant attention.

4. Time constraints and heavy workloads create stress.
   Communication in healthcare often takes place under stress and time pressures. These can lead to hurried and vague communication, which does not lend itself to full and accurate information sharing. This impediment is not easily removed, but strategies can be put in place to ensure more effective communication in spite of it.
5. Interpersonal conflict strongly affects communication within and across teams.
   When conflict is present, communication becomes closed. In the resulting frigid environment, people communicate as little as possible. Often only essential information is passed along, while general information and observations—very important to patient care—are omitted.
6. Team members may be unclear about their roles, and therefore uncertain about who is responsible in a particular situation.
   In this case, there is confusion around what to communicate and to whom. So, assumptions are made about who is the decision maker and when to speak up.

In order to overcome the factors that impede communication, two things in particular must be considered: the individuals' ability to communicate effectively (*how* they communicate), and the degree of structure applied in the situation. The ability to communicate effectively can be the more difficult, because it depends on individuals' personal style and development. The degree of structure in a situation can be addressed with the use of easily learned tools that we provide in Part II: Making It Happen.

PURE COMMUNICATION

Our species is unique in its communication challenges. Many species have well-developed and nearly foolproof communication systems. Ants, for example, have been lauded for what we think of as pure communication.

The purity of their communication is the main ingredient in their renowned teamwork. For centuries ants have been held up as an example for humans. The book of Proverbs in the Bible uses ants as an example of hard work and co-operation. The Chinese character for *ant* combines a logogram that represents *insect* with another that means *which acts properly*.

Ants are particularly impressive because as individuals they have limited brainpower, but in concert they achieve amazing things. Their engineering skills, which require considerable co-operation, are sophisticated. Underground nests are designed to be well oxygenated, and the hill on top is engineered to regulate the nest's temperature. When temperatures drop, the ants are mobilized to block the entrances with dirt; if conditions are too dry, members go out to find water and bring it back to increase the humidity. When environments change, colonies adjust by changing the number of workers allocated to various tasks. Ants work together to solve problems. They team up to create paths between the nest and a food source, retrieve dead mates, or build living bridges across swampy land. How can they be so efficient and effective?

An important strength is that they are incapable of miscommunication. They pass messages by laying chemical trails of pheromones. Their antennae gather information by picking up scents. They therefore receive information in its purest form. No perceptions or assumptions get in the way. There is no hasty or sloppy communication that causes misunderstandings, misdirection, or general confusion.[3]

Pure communication is critical to healthcare. In no other environment is clear and immediate communication so important. However, we need enhanced pure communication that allows for appropriate individual decision making, rather than requiring that one follow the trail laid by someone else, as in the case of the ants.

Pure communication in healthcare has several components:

- It is timely.
- The message and response are given with sensitivity and without negative emotion.
- Content is expressed clearly and accurately.

- It is given with a pure purpose (i.e., for the good of the patient, team, or organization).
- Messages are received in the same spirit.

Pure communication has been created if a nurse spots a potential error, does not hesitate to raise her concern due to fear of how her comment might be received, and communicates her message effectively, and if her message is received in the spirit it is intended. Pure communication is dependent on both the sender and receiver. The sender's role can be more important because the way in which the message is sent may influence the receiver's response. However, a poorly sent message does not remove the receiver's responsibility, or excuse a negative response.

Pure communication depends very much on the emotional maturity of the participants. Emotionally mature participants are self-aware; they recognize when an interaction triggers their emotions, and they are able to manage them and choose an appropriate response.

Any situation in which accuracy is important requires pure communication. This includes one-on-one or interpersonal communication, as well as more structured group situations.

Pure communication also requires that each individual take responsibility for *how* they are communicating. They must pay conscious attention to how their message might be received by the other party. In the survey of over 150 healthcare workers that we referred to earlier, 65 per cent indicated that they were frustrated by the way in which team members communicate with one another on their unit. These same respondents identified the following behaviours and practices as most important to creating effective communication on their unit:

- Positive body language, including tone of voice, facial expression, posture, and eye contact (all non-verbal cues should communicate "I'm open to hearing what you have to say")
- A belief that your opinion holds value, and that the receiver of the information is open to hearing your opinion
- Being able to share ideas without fear of consequences, retaliation, or judgment
- Being comfortable with exploring ideas and asking questions

- Effective transfer of information from person to person, which is measured by
    - The receptiveness of the receiver to hear the information
    - Clear, concise, and accurate delivery of information
    - The understanding that the message given is received as intended

The behaviours and practices described reflect one of the most critical skills in developing pure communication: dialoguing.

DIALOGUE

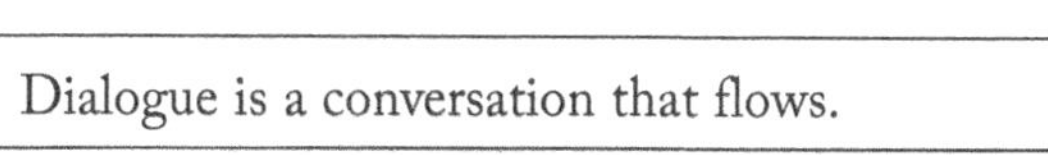
Dialogue is a conversation that flows.

Dialogue is more than a communication technique; it is the trigger for and means of maintaining connectedness. With dialogue, individuals are able to interact in ways that build shared meaning through the exploration of ideas and opinions. It makes it possible for the whole to be more than the sum of its parts. Much communication that occurs within teams is not dialogue; it is discussion that results in a collision of opinions and perceptions, which creates frustration and miscommunication.

The task-oriented, urgent world of healthcare is often more conducive to discussion than dialogue. When interaction is purely discussion, members see their primary responsibility as clearly presenting their point of view, and convincing others that their point of view is the right one.

Dialogue, on the other hand, requires a very different type of participation in which team members are committed to an effective process and best outcomes, rather than to their own point of view. The intent is to create a fully understood picture or body of knowledge from which the best decision can emerge. To communicate through dialogue, each member must clear a pathway for understanding by setting aside their assumptions, their conviction that their own position is the "right" one, and any attached emotions that could lead to defensiveness or other negative responses. Dialogue requires people to shift from telling others what they think to inquiring about what others think. Individuals must practice focused listening that comes from a sincere interest in understanding.

Dialogue does not exclude aspects of the traditional discussion mode if they are used appropriately. One still must be able to present one's opinion clearly and challenge others, but do so in a way that will not block the other person from listening and, importantly, bringing things to closure. Group dialogue is a well-managed process that ensures full understanding and consensus, but does so efficiently.

In dialogue, it is not the individual but the body of knowledge created by the group that influences people's thinking, and ultimately, the outcomes. In dialogue, critical thinking is sparked, the best outcomes are achieved, and relationships are built.

We once had the pleasure of working with a First Nations community. The members of the community were models of effective dialogue, with an exemplary ability to listen and reflect, and then speak after thoughtfully considering whether what they had to say added to the conversation. Listening was critical; but, as individual members sat quietly, and then gradually moved into consensus on what had been a divisive issue, it became clear that an essential part of the dialogue process had been reflection.

Dialogue is as important in one-on-one interactions as it is in group conversations. When asked what contributed most to her job fulfillment and her ability to do her job well, a nurse practicing on the transplant unit described an environment in which dialogue was the communication norm.

"I know that what I have to say matters," she said. "I know that I can speak up and people—the nurses, physicians, anesthesiologists, social workers, everyone—will really listen to me." She went on to share that physicians on her unit regularly ask the nurses, "What do you think?" And she added, "That makes us feel so good. There's no hierarchy, no ego. It's about giving our best to the patient, and that means tapping each team member's skills, knowledge, and perspective on how to best care for that patient. Even though I've only been practising for a year, docs still ask me what I think—it's amazing!"

Dialogue starts with questions, and culminates in the best possible results.

Recognizing the need for dialogue in shift-change reporting has led some healthcare facilities, which had previously been using a recorded audiotape report, to implement a process that includes a face-to-face report, sometimes at the bedside of the patient. Important care information can be unclear or overlooked in audiotaped reports, and without the opportunity to ask questions and probe more deeply into the patient's situation, the patient may be put at risk due to incorrect assumptions made by the healthcare professional or critical patient information being accidentally left out of the reporting. In 2000, the Joint Commission on Accreditation of Healthcare Organizations identified communication failures during shift reports as a leading cause of sentinel events in the United States. In 2006, they established a standardized approach to hand-off communication as a key component of one of the 2007 National Patient Safety Goals for U.S. hospitals. This goal emphasized the importance of allowing caregivers the opportunity to ask and respond to questions during hand-offs, including change-of-shift reports.[4]

Dialogue techniques can powerfully transform conversations inside and outside of meetings. Even if most team members haven't learned the techniques, if one or two demonstrate them well, the tone of the interaction can be changed. Other members tend to become more open and begin to mirror the behaviours of those skilled in dialogue.

Imagine how dialogue can bring about learning in adverse-events briefings. Imagine how dialogue with the patient can contribute to the best possible care and make him or her feel like a team member. Imagine how dialogue can resolve conflict. Imagine the impact on healthcare should dialogue become the norm in every facility. Getting to that point starts with everyone learning how. We include the essential behaviours and practices in the section which follows.

Open communication is essential to problem solving, which means it is the first element of high-performance healthcare that should be assessed and developed. If teams cannot communicate, they will not be able to effectively resolve issues that relate to the other six elements.

When an environment of positive, open communication is created, attitudes become more positive and the atmosphere more cheerful. As a result, not only is patient information communicated clearly and completely, but also the climate becomes one that is conducive to healing for the patient, and one that helps team members thrive.

> "The aim of argument, or of discussion, should not be victory, but progress."
>
> —Joseph Joubert

The Behaviours and Practices that Create Open and Effective Communication

Dialogue is the epitome of open and effective communication. The following requirements are the basics of good communication and the creators of dialogue.

1. Listen. Really Listen!

> "Wisdom is the reward you get for a lifetime of listening when you would have preferred to talk."
>
> —Doug Larson

Listening requires more than simply waiting for a turn to speak. Listening is choosing to truly understand what the other person is saying, and is the first step in ensuring an open two-way conversation. Listening requires setting aside judgment and any preconceived notions about the other individual and their ideas and perspectives, so that the information can be received in its purest form.

Listening requires that individuals take the following measures:

- Give their full attention to the speaker and resist using the speaker's airtime to prepare their next comments
- Silence their inner voice
- Suspend judgment
- Acknowledge the speaker's statements
- Resist interrupting the speaker

2. Respond Instead of React

Our response to another individual is likely to trigger their next response. A defensive, aggressive, or judgmental reaction invites and often receives an equally unproductive response. An opportunity for understanding and best outcomes is lost, and miscommunication and possibly conflict are generated.

Responding effectively requires that individuals take the following measures:

- Be committed to creating a positive interaction
- Be respectful in choice of words and tone of voice
- Suspend judgment
- Be self-aware

It takes self-awareness to respond effectively, particularly in stressful situations. A response includes words, tone of voice, and body language. When people are aware of the impact these have on the message being relayed, it allows them to better choose their response. Nonproductive reactions have been given no objective thought, are based primarily on emotion, and often elicit an unproductive response in the other person. Self-awareness also includes being aware of the assumptions that one holds.

3. Ask Questions and Clarify

"Seek first to understand, then to be understood."

—Stephen Covey, *The 7 Habits of Highly Effective People*

In the hurried healthcare environment, probing that is critical to understanding and accuracy can be overlooked. The practice of asking questions enriches communication in the following ways:

- Clarifying meaning
- Reducing errors
- Reducing assumptions

- Building common understanding
- Triggering new thinking and new conversation, leading to better outcomes
- Sparking new learning

Creating an environment in which people regularly ask questions of one another will not only promote better communication and fewer errors, it will promote an environment in which people trust that when an individual asks a question, it is with a positive intent. Team members comfortably adopt questioning when its use is seen as a sign of strength and confidence, as opposed to a sign of weakness or lack of competence.

4. Recap Understanding

Misunderstanding is perhaps the most dangerous communication hazard, and it can happen so easily. The receiver may be preoccupied for just a few seconds and miss an important piece without realizing it; the sender may be in a hurry or may be stressed, and may not take sufficient time to explain or to check for understanding; a cultural mix between workers can result in misunderstanding due to language differences or cultural interpretation.

A simple recap can prevent team members from leaving an interaction with information that is incomplete or an understanding that is incorrect. A recap is the repetition of the key points that need to be taken away. The recap is often done by the sender, but can also be done by the receiver to check that he or she has understood. It can be used in briefings, debriefings, staff meetings, hand-offs, and other one-on-one exchanges.

On occasion, team members are hesitant to recap for fear the recipient may feel that he or she is being talked down to. This can be prevented by statements such as, "I just want to make sure I've communicated everything well," or, for the receiver, "I just want to make sure I understand." Recaps can make a strong contribution to team effectiveness and patient safety when the team adopts them as a practice.

REFLECTION AND APPLICATION

Signs That the Open Communication Element Is Strong

Leaders can conduct a quick check of their team's communication with the following assessment. Assign a response of Yes, No, or Sometimes to each of the following questions.

Do team members...	**Yes / No / Sometimes**
...communicate with each other in a respectful manner at all times?	
...receive input from one another in an open and receptive manner?	
...communicate their point of view readily, without fear of reprisal?	
...feel free to question the decisions and actions of others regardless of their level of authority?	
...take the time to listen to one another and ask questions as needed?	
...practice the principles of effective communication?	

The open communication element requires strengthening when one or more of the above questions is rated a "Sometimes" or a "No."

Reflection and Application for Leaders

Opening the Flow of Communication

Team meetings are a good opportunity to engage in open communication and dialogue with team members, and often represent the only time for team members to ask questions and provide input on issues impacting the team and patient-care processes. Oftentimes, however, the structure, tone, and type of information shared at the meetings does not create an environment conducive to participation, leaving team members feeling

(*continued*)

disconnected and frustrated, or resulting in team members fully checking out and not participating or listening in the meeting.

Reflect on your team meetings and respond to the following statements (Yes or No):

1. Our team meetings focus just as much on group discussion as on information sharing.
2. In our team meetings, team members actively participate by asking questions and sharing input.
3. Our team meetings are seen as a productive use of time and are well attended.
4. Our team meetings are interprofessional.
5. There is positive dialogue among and between professions at our team meetings.

For any statement you responded to with a "No," review the following tips and select ones that you can implement to strengthen the communication that occurs within your meetings.

Tips:

- Reflect on the objective of your team meetings. Ensure that the team meeting and its agenda items are consistently focused on helping the team achieve its overall objective (i.e., delivering exceptional patient care).
- Make agenda items that engage team members in dialogue and require them to voice their input and opinions a priority.
- If team meetings often take the format of "information downloading," identify the items that can be shared in other ways. For example, some information can be passed on via e-mail, thereby freeing up time in meetings to focus on items that spark participation.
- To encourage participation, consider breaking the team into smaller groups for discussion purposes during the meeting.
- Invite team members to develop a set of meeting agreements that describe the behaviours and practices they believe are essential to

(*continued*)

effective communication during meetings. Ask them to complete the following sentence: "In order to have more productive meetings with full participation, we need to..."

- Hold regular interprofessional team meetings for the purpose of identifying ways to strengthen the team, improve the quality of patient care, and develop more interprofessional collaboration.

Reflection and Application for Everyone

1. Enhancing Pure Communication

Pure and open communication starts with each individual. Set aside at least 10 minutes of quiet time to reflect on the following.

1. Do you recall leaving an interaction knowing that something is expected of you but unsure what it is? Would it have been useful to ask for more information? If so, what prevented you from doing so?
2. Do you recall leaving an interaction with a negative feeling such as anger, frustration, annoyance, lower self-esteem, or inadequacy? What caused this outcome? Could you have done anything to manage the interaction differently, thereby changing or influencing the outcome? What can you do in future interactions to prevent a similar outcome?

2. Creating Dialogue

> "Reflection and inquiry skills provide a foundation for dialogue."
>
> —Peter Senge

Take a few minutes to check your dialoguing skills by answering these questions.

In one-on-one conversations and in meetings do I

- Do more asking or more telling?
- Do more "real" listening than talking?
- Probe to ensure that I fully understand a point?
- Listen to comments from others who may disagree with my perspective before jumping in to explain why my position is right?

(continued)

- Reflect on and thoughtfully consider what others are saying?
- Make an effort to recognize and challenge my own assumptions?

If you are an appointed leader, when you are in one-on-one conversations and in meetings, ask yourself:

- Do I model effective dialoguing skills?
- Am I being completely honest with myself in answering these questions?

If you answered a confident "Yes" to each of these questions, your dialoguing skills are in good shape and you make a good example for others. If you responded "No" to any of the questions, or if you perhaps hesitated over your answers, these questions represent *growth opportunities* (GOs) for you.

3. Responding Effectively

Reflect on each of the following quotations and ask yourself:

- How might this apply to me?
- Does it suggest a GO for me?

> "Every person in this life has something to teach me—and as soon as I accept that, I open myself to truly listening."
>
> —Catherine Doucette

> "Between stimulus and response, man has the freedom to choose."
>
> —Viktor Frankl

5

Change Compatibility
From Rigidity to Flexibility

As we write this book, the oncology team at the Niagara Health System (NHS) is preparing for a substantial change. After over 20 years of working in their current facility, they are moving to a new state-of-the-art centre that will provide their patients with a greater number of on-site services and more modern amenities that will no doubt enhance the patient experience and quality of care. A change of this magnitude comes with a number of challenges, most importantly ensuring the team is prepared to manage the transition so that the changes have no negative impact on the team's ability to provide the best care possible. The success of the move will ultimately be determined neither by the team's ability to implement a project plan nor by the leader's ability to identify and manage logistical issues. While these are important, success will be driven in great part by the team's attitude toward the change, members' willingness to be flexible and adaptable during this period of change, and their commitment to ensuring the change is a success.

The move to the new facility is the perfect analogy for change. Change of any kind is the process of moving to a new state of things. Whether it is a change in policies, procedures, or protocols, a change in technology and equipment, or a change in how we communicate and interact with our team members, change involves moving from a known state to an unknown one; it requires letting go of the old and embracing the new.

Successful organizational change can only happen through people. When initiating a change process, the first priority of the effective leader is to support the team in developing as positive an attitude as possible toward the change. In some instances, such as site closings and layoffs, what is generally thought of as a positive attitude is unlikely. Enthusiasm will be difficult to engender. But well developed teams are able to manage their attitude to change that may not be of their choosing and do their best to effectively carry out their role in its implementation. It is seldom the logistical issues that derail an initiative. More often, it is the ability or inability of the team to come together in a receptive and adaptive manner that will determine whether the change initiative is a success. Whether or not the team is able to achieve this depends on its *change compatibility*. Change compatibility includes responsiveness to change, an ability to effectively implement change, and an ability to make change stick. The degree of receptivity is most critical, as it also affects whether the change will be effectively implemented and whether the change takes.

CHANGE RESPONSIVENESS

In many cases, the way in which a team responds to change is a direct reflection of how well the members are working together. The oncology team at Niagara Health System, which was undergoing a major change that was not of their making, could have presented any one of three possible responses: rigid, limp, or flexible.

The Rigid Response

When rigidity is displayed, the team or a number of its members dig in their collective heels and focus energy and attitude on the reasons why the change is a bad idea. If it is within the team's power, the change may be derailed, and if not, negative attitudes and lack of support for the change may hinder effective implementation. In any case, rigid responses are strong and emotional, and create a distraction that can prevent members from being able to give the very best of themselves to their patients and their colleagues.

Rigidity increases when a team is in a state of unease, which can settle in when there is lack of collaboration, trust, and cohesiveness. Change frequently does not stick. If it has not been hard-wired into team processes it fades away as members gradually and quietly ignore it and revert to the old way of doing things.

The Limp Response

When there is a limp response, members pay lip service to the change. They choose not to rock the boat, so although they never resist the change, neither do they actively embrace it. The success of the change is weakened by lack of commitment to it; it is on the bottom of the team's priority list. A limp response can prove to be even more destructive to a change process than a rigid response, because the lack of support is not as evident as when there is blatant resistance, and is therefore not addressed.

A limp response frequently puts change, which is meant to be maintained by the team, at risk. If a limp response is the norm, even change that members have initiated themselves is likely to fail. Comments such as, "Didn't we put a new process in place a while ago that was supposed to look after that?" are common in teams in which the limp response has become the norm. When new initiatives are put in place, they often fizzle out quickly due to a lack of urgency, commitment, and appropriate structures. A group of nurses discussing morning huddles, a positive routine that had disappeared, acknowledged that they weren't sure what had happened to them. "We used to have them every morning and they were great. Come to think of it, I'm not sure why or even when we stopped having them," one nurse commented. Too often when the limp response is the norm, good things are lost.

In teams that display either a rigid or a limp response to change, members suffer from the stress of working in a negative environment and perhaps, in addition, from fear of the change. *Will I be able to handle the added responsibilities? Can I adjust? Will there be a place for me?* This stress, if maintained over a period of time, can affect individuals physically and emotionally, and eventually create problems for the team in the form of increased absenteeism, conflict, low morale, and a drop in quality of care.

The Flexible Response

> "If you don't like something, change it. If you can't change it, change your attitude."
>
> —Maya Angelou

Teams that present a flexible response embrace change. They may look for more information about a change decision in order to have a better understanding, but whether or not they fully agree with the change, they commit to making it work.

Flexibility doesn't imply a lack of emotion or a lack of fear. Flexible teams do not necessarily have any more courage or fewer emotions than those with limp or rigid responses. The difference is how their fears and emotions are managed. Flexible teams neither ignore nor overly inflate emotions and fears. These are openly talked about and addressed so that the teams can find strategies for effectively managing them.

A flexible response comes more easily to some teams than others. In well-developed, high-performance teams, maturity, energy, and enthusiasm allow members to deal effectively with whatever comes their way. A high-performance team is not threatened by change. Its change compatibility element is strong. In addition, the team's strength in the other essential elements is strong, which contributes to its embracing and effectively managing change. Members are not wasting energy on conflict; they know they can trust one another; there is shared leadership so they have a voice in change; and members support one another and share the load of change. They have created a team culture conducive to effective change.

However, a team's change compatibility can be strengthened even if the team is not yet a fully high-performing team.

Avoiding Rigid and Limp Responses

> "Change is a threat when done to me, but an opportunity when done by me."
>
> —Rosabeth Moss Kanter, "Seven Truths about Change to Lead By and Live By"

Resistance is most likely to occur when change is seen as being imposed, is viewed as threatening, or is not believed in or understood.

When team members feel that change is being forced upon them rather than feeling empowered to own the change, stress and negativity abound, trust is put at risk, and the change itself seldom materializes as originally envisioned. Ownership requires an opportunity to understand the benefits of the change and how it will affect members, to acknowledge and deal with fears, and to give input that will be used to support the change.

The leaders of the oncology team at Niagara Health System recognized that engaging team members in the change process was critical to the success of the team and to the team's well-being. Members were assigned to smaller groups in which there was full opportunity for participation. Members shared their feelings about the change and identified what they believed team leaders and members needed to do to best manage the change. They discussed the benefits the move would bring to their patients, while at the same time acknowledged they had fears of the unknown. But they knew they could manage their fears by relying on one another for support and by choosing to believe that their leaders would do their best to support them and keep them informed along the way.

Full and transparent communication is a key part of an effective participation process. The more sensitive the issue, the better the communication process needs to be. If there is concern about how a change will affect staff or patients, emotions can run high and rigidity can quickly set in. An understanding of why the change is being implemented, and plans to manage any possible downsides, are critical to the team's receptivity.

Ideal communication is early, planned, positive, participative, and ongoing.

A conversation between a group of nurses over lunch reflected a lack of understanding about an upcoming change. They were discussing the recent change to their change-of-shift reporting process. The process was to be changed from a pre-recorded audiotaped report to a bedside report that required the nurses to move from one patient to the next, reviewing the patient's case. The discussion at the table focused primarily on what were seen as the downsides of the new process, such as issues associated with the impact on the patient's privacy and the extra time and work it would take compared to the original reporting process. There was no discussion about the benefits of the new process, such as how bedside reporting creates the opportunity to engage the patient and provides the opportunity to ask more questions and to have a greater dialogue, which could result in better patient care.

It was evident that there was a lack of understanding among the nurses as to why the new process had been initiated, and frustrations about how the change would take place. There appeared to have been little opportunity for the nurses to give input during the decision-making process, or to get information about the rationale behind the decision. From the tone of the discussion, it was evident that the transition to the new bedside reporting process would not be as smooth as it could be, and that it would result in a greater number of bumps in the road and higher levels of frustration and stress than there needed to be.

It is highly preferable to prevent the kind of reaction the nurses experienced by demonstrating early effective communication. However, if that hasn't happened, the leader can still spark increased receptivity to the change by providing an opportunity for communication and productive discussion that includes how the team can best make the change work.

STRENGTHENING CHANGE COMPATIBILITY

Resistance is most likely to occur when change is seen as being imposed, is viewed as threatening, or is not believed in or understood.

---

1. Create Member Engagement and Let the Team Own the Change

The change compatibility element is strengthened when the team develops the habit of objectively examining important or dramatic change, and developing strategies for implementing or dealing with it. With practice the team comes to respond rather than react to change. The sense of engagement and teamwork that is created can boost energy and attitude and allow individuals to more quickly accept change.

Engagement is successful when dialogue is structured effectively and facilitates honest communication. It is much easier to facilitate a productive meeting when good structure is in place. When emotions are high as a result of change, the outcome can be a breakdown of structure, which turns an opportunity for growth into a negative session rife with venting and complaining. You can provide structure by building a framework based on the following questions:

- What are the benefits of the change?
- What are the downsides of the change?
- If the downsides seem to outweigh the benefits, do we have the power to stop or alter the change, or to request that it is re-examined?
    - If the answer is no, what do we need to do in order to demonstrate a positive attitude, even though it is not a change we would have chosen?
- What do we have to do to ensure the change is a success?
- How can we support one another through the change process?
- What do we need from our leaders to effectively implement and manage the change?

An effective process results in the team identifying specific commitments to action that clearly articulate how they will best implement the change and support one another through it. High performance teams that successfully implement change, regularly review their commitments and hold one another accountable to them.

2. Make Change Stick

Change that sticks has "stay" plans attached to it.

Teams with strong change compatibility do not allow a change to gradually fade away. Poor execution of good ideas is frequently an organizational issue. Team members spend time identifying opportunities for change, and either nothing happens, or change is initiated but doesn't take. The apparently small initiatives that are introduced and maintained by the team are particularly at risk.

One such small change was a suggestion box that was introduced into a healthcare unit as a method of increasing the input from team members. All members had thought it was a good idea, but within a short time the box disappeared. No one could remember who had been assigned to collect the suggestions, and no one could remember when the box had disappeared. The suggestion box could have been a catalyst for important change. Instead, it simply disappeared both from the unit and from the consciousness of team members. Teams waste a lot of time developing initiatives that don't stick.

Change that sticks has "stay" plans attached to it. Perhaps this stay plan is in the form of a change champion, which Kurt Lewin dubbed a "stay agent." This individual is responsible for ensuring that the change happens and stays in place as envisioned, and alerts the team to anything that needs to be revisited or shored up. At the very least, the team must follow up on its commitments or action items assigned to members through the engagement process as discussed in the first step above.

3. Set an Example

The leader's attitude toward change and his or her expectations of team members strongly influence the team's change compatibility. Leaders who have teams that demonstrate change compatibility set an example by presenting a positive, objective attitude to change. The team leader establishes clear expectations of change behaviour, and will not accept a negative attitude toward a change. The leader welcomes discussion and encourages team members to voice concerns, but ensures that the discussion does not get bogged down with complaints about why the change won't work. Instead, he or she focuses on how the team will make the change work.

4. Strengthen the Team

Leaders whose teams face a major change are wise to check the fitness level of the team and, if need be, put initiatives and practices in place to strengthen it. This requires strengthening not only the team's change compatibility, but all of the elements of a high-performance team. Although all elements together determine the team's fitness, the elements of open communication, climate, and cohesiveness are particularly important to ensuring the team is able to continue to provide exceptional care throughout the change process.

Even the best teams need support in preparing for significant change. The director of the Niagara Health System's oncology program recognized the need for her team to be functioning at its best and for the team to be as cohesive as possible as they prepared for the transition to the new facility. Recognizing the stress that the impending move could have on her team, the director took a proactive approach by initiating a team development process designed to leverage her team's strengths and actively address any areas of weakness. The director recognized that if her team was not flexible and functioning at a level of high performance, not only would the successful transition to the new facility be put at risk, but the well-being of her staff and their patients would be as well.

High-performance teams demonstrate their change compatibility by

- Being open to new ideas
- Taking a positive attitude toward change with which they may not agree, but over which they have no control
- Looking for productive change opportunities, but not getting caught up in change for change's sake
- Implementing change effectively
- Putting structures and processes in place to ensure change sticks
- Taking time during a change process, even when they believe they have no time, to check that members are coping effectively

We find that Rosabeth Moss Kanter's statement that "change is a threat when done to me, but an opportunity when done by me" consistently holds true[1]. Flexible teams and their leaders know that fears and emotions are very real, and if they are not listened to and sincerely acknowledged, they can have a detrimental impact on the team's ability to positively respond to the change. When emotions are ignored, teams are more likely to react impulsively rather than respond productively.

Flexible teams also know there is real value in the voicing of opinions. When leaders solicit opinions and really listen to them, team members may share perspectives that bring to light potential risks that may not otherwise have been uncovered. Through the NHS oncology team development process, team members have had the opportunity to voice their opinions, to identify where they believe the team's strengths lie, and to determine where real progress needs to be made in order to improve the team's effectiveness. They are given the opportunity to voice their fears and concerns regarding the impending move, and to communicate what they need from their leaders and colleagues in order to confidently and effectively transition to the new facility.

REFLECTION AND APPLICATION

Signs That the Change Compatibility Element Is Strong

Leaders can conduct a quick check of their team's change compatibility with the following assessment. Assign a response of Yes, No, or Sometimes to each of the following questions.

Do team members...	Yes / No / Sometimes
...make themselves open to new ideas?	
...take a positive attitude toward change (regardless of whether they agree with it or not)?	
...implement change effectively?	
...effectively support one another through change?	
...ensure that change sticks once it is implemented?	

The change compatibility element requires strengthening when one or more of the above questions is rated a "Sometimes" or a "No."

Reflection and Application for Leaders

1. Reflect on an Upcoming Change

Set aside 15 minutes to reflect on the following two quotations:

"People don't resist change. They resist being changed."—Peter Senge
"When people plan the battle, they don't battle the plan."—Unknown

(continued)

What thoughts do these quotations trigger that apply to your upcoming change?

List what you will do to help ensure that the change is well implemented within your team.

2. Plan to Use Communication Well During the Change Process

Reflect on an upcoming change and consider how you will incorporate the following recommendations for effective communication during the change process.

Ideal communication is

- Early. If you don't present the facts early in the process, the rumour mill will fill the information gap. Best to get the right information out first than to try to correct misinformation and already-formed opinions and perceptions.
- Planned. It is important to think ahead before rushing into a meeting in which you will be discussing a change. What are the issues that will be on staff members' minds? How can you productively address them? How are team members likely to respond? What information is essential to them? If you don't have the essential information at hand, how can you get it?
- Positive. When the change brings with it obvious benefits, share them effectively. In particular, emphasize how the change will make life better for the staff and the patient. However, not every change is going to be seen as positive. Indeed, some changes may not be positive at all. So how do you present them positively? To maintain a positive perspective through difficult change, the leader should do the following:
  - Present the facts
  - Allow a reasonable but managed time period for venting (if team members don't vent during the meeting, they will do so elsewhere and negativity will grow)
  - Express his or her personal commitment to making the change work and to supporting the team
  - Communicate his or her expectation that the team will also be supportive

(*continued*)

You might say something like, "I know this raises some concerns, but it is our job to make this change work as effectively as possible. I intend to do just that and I know I can count on you to work with me in making this happen. Let's talk about how we can best make this work." Leaders who have built a team and have earned the team's respect will find that their team members will respond to their call.

- Participative. Decide how team members can participate in change decisions. If the decision has already been made and has been handed fully developed to the team, consider how members might assist in decisions about its implementation. At the very least, if the change is significant, invite discussion about how the members can support one another through the change.
- Ongoing. Too often a major change is announced and then nothing further is heard for some time. Team members can become uneasy wondering what is happening—or not happening—and again the rumour mill will fill the void. Keep members informed as much as possible on an ongoing basis.

Refection and Application for Everyone

Consider your most natural response to change.

- Is your first response to a change you do not fully agree with rigid, limp, or flexible?
- How do you tend to demonstrate that response?
- Did you identify any behaviours in yourself that are not responsive or helpful in the successful implementation of change?

Jot down any behaviours you will change.

6

Team Members' Contribution

The Sum of the Parts

In team development, the aim is synergy in which the whole is greater than the sum of its parts. This, however, does not negate the importance of the parts; the stronger the parts, the greater the team potential.

Strong members fully contribute to the team. It is no longer enough to fulfill one's individual role competently. Fully contributing team members not only have the necessary clinical skills and knowledge, but also recognize that they share responsibility for ensuring that everyone works effectively together to provide the best care possible.

Fully contributing team members:

- Appreciate and support their colleagues
- Focus on what is best for the team and patient rather than themselves
- Take responsibility for their interpersonal relations and communication
- Take initiative to solve issues on their own
- Readily share information and knowledge
- Recognize when team members require assistance, and respond whenever possible
- Spot and embrace learning opportunities

This may sound like an onerous list when the day-to-day life on the unit is already full, but in a high-performance team in which generous gestures are reciprocated, and positive behaviour is the norm and appreciated, these practices come naturally. A utopia? No, this is the way we are meant to work. Somehow, too many groups have fallen off the high-performance road and haven't made a concerted effort to get back on. The longer the leader takes to steer the team back on course, the tougher the task becomes.

The old adage that a team is as strong as its weakest link holds true. When a team member is perceived as one who doesn't share the load, doesn't take ownership of issues, and doesn't help fellow team members, interpersonal and professional relationships are affected. Communication and trust break down, which can then have a ripple effect on the team's morale. Negative and unproductive behaviour can become contagious if team members begin to see it as accepted. This is particularly true when team leaders fail to reward and acknowledge positive behaviour. Individuals may begin to wonder, "What's the point?" which can cause a downward spiral into mediocrity and complacency, and negatively impact patient care and the staff experience. When team members don't share the load, stress and even burnout increase.

A nurse in an emergency department shared the following comment: "I feel like not everyone is pulling their weight. When asking others to help, you get a lot of resistance. If we would just take the time to help one another out and stop saying, 'That's not my job,' it would make a world of difference."

Fully contributing team members share responsibility for ensuring that everyone works effectively together to provide the best care possible.

BRINGING OUT THE BEST IN PEOPLE

The leader plays an important role in strengthening team members' contribution. It is when members feel good about themselves that they are best able to contribute to the team. Although feeling good about oneself is ultimately the individual's own responsibility, the leader plays an important role in supporting members in reaching that state.

It might seem that making people feel good about themselves would be an obvious leadership priority. However, there are many reasons why leaders may fail to ensure that this happens consistently in every team across every healthcare organization. For example, leaders often believe they are already doing everything they can to ensure people are at their best, but the members of the teams they lead might not think it's enough. Busy leaders may intend to do what is required to make each team member feel good, but overlook the little things, such as stopping to say good morning, or taking the time to ask a team member for his or her opinion. Many leaders simply do not understand what is required to make people feel good about themselves, and others believe that making people feel good means being too soft. They believe that being nice translates into accepting excuses and mediocrity.

Making people feel good about themselves is just the opposite to accepting mediocrity. When people know their performance is lacking, they seldom feel good about themselves. They may put up a front that looks like confidence, or even arrogance, but when one digs deeper, one finds a less-than-self-satisfied individual. It is our nature as human beings to want to achieve and be recognized for our achievements. The type of recognition that people desire may differ, but everyone needs to know that they count and that they are making a contribution. It is an important part of valuing oneself.

The power of making people feel good about themselves was dramatically demonstrated in a conversation that we overheard during a reception we attended in a corporate office. It was winter in Toronto, and there had been a great deal of snow. Two fellows were making the kind of small talk often made when sharing a drink with someone you don't know particularly well. One man asked the other where he lived, and the second man responded that he was from Oshawa, about 50 kilometres east of Toronto. This meant that he had a long commute on Highway 401, the main artery leading into the city.

"Boy," said the first fellow. "You must want to find a job closer to home, particularly when the weather is as bad as it's been."

"No way," was the response. "Mark [his manager] makes it worth the drive every day."

What a compliment! We later investigated to find out exactly what Mark did every day to create such a level of commitment in his employees. We found that Mark demonstrated the following practices:

- Showed a sincere personal interest in people
- Created high expectations
- Coached and supported individuals in meeting those expectations

- Recognized people's successes and broadcast those successes
- Always made time (The needs of the people who reported to him were always his first priority—no matter what! He knew if they felt good about themselves and excelled that everything else would fall into place.)

A nurse in an adult medical/surgical unit described the following characteristics, which indicated to her that her manager was a strong and caring leader:

- Strove to understand the perspectives of those working on the front line, regardless of how busy she was
- Encouraged staff to come to her with ideas and to share opinions
- Offered to help when she could, and in doing so demonstrated the importance of supporting one another

Busy leaders often don't recognize that team members notice their positive behaviours and practices, nor do they realize the extent to which these then influence team attitude and morale.

The fastest way to change others is to change yourself.

When the leader takes the initiative to recognize and appreciate the contributions and skill sets of each team member, team members will begin to follow their lead and demonstrate the same generosity of spirit, so that it becomes part of "the way we do things around here."

People feel good about themselves when:

- They believe they are part of something special.
- They are listened to and know they have been heard.
- They are growing, when they have the opportunity to stretch themselves and achieve higher levels of performance.
- They are achieving and know they are delivering the best possible patient care.
- Their contribution is recognized.
- "People first" is a motto that keeps the leader's teamwork compass pointed true north.

DEVELOP THE TEAM, DEVELOP ITS MEMBERS

Leaders who embark on a team development process are at the same time supporting the development of the members. Once a high-performance team is developed, team members have an increased sense of ownership for their own development and are able to support one another's growth. Team spirit has been sparked, and there is an increased pride in the team and its service. When people feel pride in being members, they make a greater effort to ensure they contribute in the best way possible. When the team is developed, trust and more effective communication allows members to give—and, very importantly, receive—feedback, which triggers personal growth.

Does every individual who is part of a team development process become a positive, fully contributing team member? Not necessarily. Very negative, unhappy individuals sometimes cling to old behaviours like a security blanket. The greatest risk is not that a member will fail to grow sufficiently, but that other team members will use the nonproductive behaviour of that individual as an excuse for not changing their own behaviour. "This will never work because *they* will never change" is a lament that can become a dangerous common theme if it is not quickly curtailed.

The best way to bring difficult individuals on board is for other team members to use the learning they gain through the team development process to respond differently to these people, remembering that "the fastest way to change others is to change yourself." When recalcitrant individuals discover that old behaviours have lost their power, and they have no base of support, they too begin to change.

CREATING INCREASED CONTRIBUTION THROUGH PASSION

> "Purpose may point you in the right direction but it is passion that propels you."
>
> —Travis McAshan

Passion provides the energy and focus that makes positive change happen. Leaders can't lead if they haven't committed to a destination. If a leader does not believe that "getting there" is important, that the journey itself will be exciting and fulfilling, the members he or she leads soon become automatons.

Admittedly, passion doesn't flare at the flip of a switch. If the challenge seems too great, or if people around us project negativism, bringing forth the passion can be difficult. However, it is far from impossible if you are committed to making things better. Every leader is capable of getting to passion and accomplishing great things as a result.

Passion can be kindled by

- Focusing on the positives that are so often buried under the challenges
- Imagining a better world—whether it is the world of the unit, the organization, or simply an even better healthcare world—and maintaining fanatical focus on that vision
- By coming into work every day with a sense of anticipation, with a sparkle in the eye—even if these things have to be consciously generated

A "fake it till you make it" attitude may be necessary to the development of passion. Commitment is critical to developing increased team member contribution, and passion makes that commitment come much more easily. When commitment is consistent, it is contagious.

Passion provides the energy and focus that makes positive change happen.

REFLECTION AND APPLICATION

Signs That the Team Members' Contribution Element Is Strong

Leaders can conduct a quick check of their team members' contribution with the following assessment. Assign a response of Yes, No, or Sometimes to each of the following questions.

Do team members...	**Yes / No / Sometimes**
...take initiative to put forth ideas and concerns?	
...take initiative to do what needs to be done without being asked?	
...take ownership for solving issues?	
...share the load?	
...share knowledge?	
...keep each other informed?	
...take responsibility for managing their interpersonal relationships?	
...embrace learning opportunities?	
...actively participate?	
...demonstrate commitment to the team's goals and values?	
...look for opportunities to improve care practice/service delivery?	

The team members' contribution element requires strengthening when one or more of the above questions is rated a "Sometimes" or a "No."

Reflection and Application for Leaders

Generate Passion

If you don't already feel the passion for a new healthcare world coursing through you, start with some visualization. Imagine yourself as a passionate leader who approaches every day with enthusiasm, and answer the following questions:

- What would be different?
- How would you behave differently?

(continued)

- Would you feel differently at the end of the day, and if so how?
- Would you feel differently at the beginning of the day, and if so how?
- How would your team members behave and respond?
- And, ultimately, how would the patient experience be different?

Reflection and Application for Everyone

Reflect on Your Contribution

Reflection, as we have advocated throughout this book, is essential to growth and superior decisions. Reflection is particularly valuable for personal development and for ensuring that you are making a strong contribution to all of your teams and relationships.

In this reflection activity we offer you several quotations that should trigger your thinking about your own attitude and behaviours. The key is not to skim them too quickly. Pause at each for a few moments and search within yourself, asking, "Is there a message here for me? Is there an opportunity within that message that I must grasp?"

When you discover a message, jot it down along with a personal commitment to action that describes what you will do differently.

This reflection can also be used with teams by setting aside 20 minutes at a team meeting to review each of the quotes and discuss them as a team.

"I've always believed that a lot of the trouble in the world would disappear if we were talking to each other instead of about each other."—Ronald Reagan

"What we do see depends mainly on what we look for."—Sir John Lubbock

"Our task . . . is not to fix blame for the past, but to fix the course for the future."—John F. Kennedy

"Anger is an acid that can do more harm to the vessel in which it stands than to anything on which it is poured."—Gandhi

"It's not the load that breaks you down, it's the way you carry it."—Lou Holtz

"The quality of a person's life is in direct proportion to their commitment to excellence, regardless of their chosen field of endeavour." —Vince Lombardi

"The only limit to your impact is your imagination and commitment." —Anthony Robbins

7

Shared Leadership
The Path to Empowered Team Members

There is no greater compliment than asking someone for their opinion on an important matter—other than, of course, handing the decision entirely over to them. When the element of *shared leadership* is strong, the leader employs both of these practices.

Traditionally, teams have been leader-centered groups in which members turn to the leader to solve problems, whether related to tasks or interpersonal relationships. The leader keeps things in motion, motivates, ensures that things get done, and makes most of the decisions.

As team members become more involved in decision making, and take on more responsibility and accountability, the team develops shared leadership, and the leader moves out of the centre of the team circle to the perimeter, an equal team member with a slightly different role.

Shared leadership depends on the leader letting go and team members stepping up and taking on more.

When shared leadership is strong, decisions, particularly those affecting the staff, department, or unit, are shared; everyone is in the know because there is generous dissemination of information. The aim of a team with shared leadership is to have members work as autonomously as possible, and to enable individuals to feel empowered to make decisions within their own areas of expertise. Shared leadership depends on both the leader and the team members. The leader must let go, and team members must step up and take over.

LETTING GO

For the leader, sharing leadership means moving from the centre of the circle. It means that he or she no longer has to be the hub—holding the team together, solving all of the problems, and making all of the decisions. "But then what is my job?" one newly appointed leader asked. That uncertainty is precisely why some managers have not become facilitative, empowering *leaders.* Historically, healthcare managers were required to focus on the administrative and managerial responsibilities that came with their jobs, and little attention was given to leadership that entailed empowering others. Max De Pree, in his book *Leadership is an Art*, defines the art of leadership as "liberating people to do what is required of them." People are liberated when each team member has the opportunity to fully participate, is empowered to make decisions, and is an equal member of the team in that their input is both valued and used whenever possible. For this to happen, however, the leader must learn to let go.

Prescribing a solution can be tempting for a leader, especially in healthcare where time is a rare commodity, and where, although this is quickly changing, directing and telling has been the historically dominant communication and management approach. Healthcare managers wear many different hats on any given day. They are firefighters, addressing the issue of the moment and working to solve a number of unexpected challenges throughout the day. They are expert jugglers, managing different priorities, patients, and team members at once. And they are high-wire artists, managing a number of different personalities and pressures—whether they are the challenges and pressures from above or from individual team members—all the while navigating the politics and hierarchy of a complex system. It is no wonder, then, that many of these leaders have developed the habit of simply reacting like a batter on a baseball mound, hitting each ball as it is thrown to them. This too can be stressful, because you don't always get a home run or even a base hit; sometimes you strike out. But you just have to be there and the ball comes to you.

Shared leadership requires that the leader toss some of the balls to the team. This not only empowers team members, but also frees the leader to dedicate more time to other important leadership responsibilities, such as developing the team and coaching individuals, working to remove any organizational issues that might be hindering the team, developing key relationships with other teams and leaders, developing and putting forward new ideas for organizational improvement, reflecting on the team and the department or unit, and planning for improvement. A unit manager could be less at his or her desk and more present on the floor observing his or her team in action, "feeling" the mood and checking the patient experience.

Besides fear of letting go of an easy-to-understand known, some leaders resist sharing leadership because they haven't had the opportunity to learn how. And still others do things themselves because it seems quicker and easier than coaching someone else to.

We recently had the opportunity to work with a group of nursing coordinators who readily talked about the challenges of being the "go-to" people for unit issues. In their units, team members trusted that the coordinator was able to solve unit problems, especially issues relating to the coordination of the unit and patient flow, and so the tendency on the part of the nursing coordinator was often to take on the issues themselves instead of delegating back to the individual. The temptation to do so was strong: it appeared to save time, allowed the coordinators to maintain control, and let them demonstrate their ability to solve problems and help others. But they also acknowledged the downsides. Failure to delegate led to a heavier workload and, for some, the feeling that they had to have all of the answers was a stress inducer. Not involving team members in decision making hindered the development of the members' critical thinking and lessened empowerment and engagement—all crucial to team effectiveness. They concluded that more letting go was essential.

The many leaders who practice shared leadership know that, when the shared leadership element is strong, team members not only develop a higher sense of self-worth and enjoy much greater job satisfaction, but they also provide superior patient care.

"Great leaders create great teams. Do not make compromises about leadership."

—Michelle DiEmanuele, President and CEO of Credit Valley Hospital

---

SHARING DECISION MAKING: THE BASICS

Leaders who are newly appointed or just beginning to develop a shared-leadership style may be tripped up if they're missing one or two basics, particularly about a shared decision-making process.

Sharing decisions and giving team members increased autonomy requires first some thoughtful decision making on the part of the leader. The leader's first consideration is *when* to involve staff in a decision. He or she must decide if the participation process would result in any of the following benefits:

- **Increased quality of the decision:** In this case the leader recognizes that staff may have important knowledge, information, or experience, which may contribute to a better decision.
- **Increased sense of empowerment among team members:** This can happen only if those invited to participate have something of substance to contribute. Participation for the sake of participation is not empowering.
- **Fully informed team members:** In major decisions that will be implemented or must be embraced by the staff, productive participation in the decision-making process can provide a greater understanding of what will need to be done. This leads to a smooth, time-saving implementation of the decision.

The next consideration is *who* to involve. Everyone can't always be involved, and the leader must consider which members' knowledge and experience is most critical to the best decision.

The final consideration is the level of influence at which members will be contributing. There are four levels of influence, as outlined in Figure 7.1. The leader may unilaterally make the decision without input from team members. The leader may invite input from team members, but will ultimately make the decision if there are other considerations outside of the team's influence that must be taken into account. The decision making could be a consensus decision with leader and members contributing to and agreeing on the decision. (For a step-by-step approach to reaching a consensus, please see Chapter 11: Facilitation: The Skill that Determines the Success of the Process.) Or, at the highest level of influence, the leader will hand the decision over to the members of their team.

4. Team members decide without the leader.

3. Consensus: Team member(s) and leader decide together.

2. Leader decides with input from team members.

1. Leader decides.

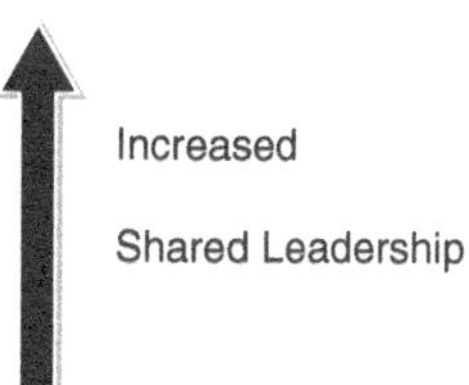

Figure 7.1: Levels of Influence

In developing shared leadership and increasing participation in the decision-making process, it is essential that both the leader and team are aware of which level they are participating at.

Potential Pitfalls of Sharing Decision Making

Pitfalls can result from the following three misconceptions regarding shared leadership:

- Misconception #1: Shared Leadership = Democratic rule
- Misconception #2: Shared Leadership = Compromise, and is designed to keep most of the people happy
- Misconception #3: Shared Leadership = Everyone has the right to be involved in every decision

When these misconceptions become operational, leaders frequently feel damned if they do and damned if they don't. The staff will be frustrated if their input is not invited, and equally frustrated if their advice is not followed. The following outcomes will result when any one of the above misconceptions is in place:

- **Staff frustration:** After giving input to decisions, staff members are frustrated because they see no evidence that their input was used. "Why ask us if they have already made up their minds, anyway?" is a common complaint. When this occurs, there is a risk of negatively impacting team member participation, making individuals less likely to contribute ideas and opinions going forward because they believe the leader is simply going through the motions of sharing leadership. Some leaders do not fully understand that it is not the participation process that is empowering, but knowing that one has made a substantive contribution.

- **Lack of support for the decision:** In many instances, a negative reaction to a decision and the resulting lack of support is the result of the leader not clarifying the participants' level of influence, or, more specifically, how their input will be used. If other factors outside of the team will influence the decision, it is important to be clear in communicating to members that their input is valued and will be carefully considered, but that the final decision may or may not reflect the input given. If a leader explains the factors that will influence a decision, the team will not feel frustrated when the final outcome does not match their perspective.

  A lab manager decided that he wanted his team to increase their participation in decision making, believing that this would increase team morale and commitment. He and his supervisors made a consistent effort over the next six months to solicit opinions from employees regarding decisions impacting the department and staff. By the sixth month, employees were frustrated rather than uplifted and motivated, and their morale had dropped. Management was equally frustrated, and concluded that involving the team in decision making didn't work. It was a lose-lose scenario.

  The team frustration stemmed from the many decisions that did not "go their way" after their having spent considerable time providing input. Their unrealistic expectations arose because no one had explained specifically how their input would be used, or how the decision would ultimately be made. There had also been no information sharing, once the final decisions were made, as to what factors contributed to the decisions.
- **Poor quality decisions:** When the goal of including individuals in the decision-making process is to keep the peace and ensure the team is happy, there is a great risk of compromise, which will result in less than optimal decision making.

Encouraging Team Member Participation in Shared Leadership

The second component of shared leadership is the willingness of team members to step up and take on more responsibility and accountability for the success of the team. There are a number of leadership skills and practices that can encourage team members to share leadership, including influencing, empowering, and coaching techniques. But most importantly team members will be more committed to taking on greater responsibility for team issues once they have begun to experience shared leadership and are rewarded by seeing that their added contribution makes a difference. More than anything, most people want to make a difference.

In Chapter 12: Leader as Coach, we describe a coaching process that can be used, in the moment and on the job, to encourage team members to think critically and take ownership of solving issues, rather than relegating issues to the leader. This chapter gives leaders the tools to toss the ball back to team members so that they can hit a home run on their own, but with support and guidance from the leader as needed.

REFLECTION AND APPLICATION

Signs That the Shared Leadership Element Is Strong

Leaders can conduct a quick check of their team's shared leadership with the following assessment. Assign a response of Yes, No, or Sometimes to each of the following questions.

Do team leaders...	Yes / No / Sometimes
...show team members that their input is valued?	
...seek input from team members on a regular basis?	
...use input from team members whenever possible?	
...empower team members to leverage their experience and skills to solve problems on their own?	
...empower team members to make decisions within their own areas of expertise?	
...keep team members well informed (in a timely manner) of decisions and information that affect them, their team, and their department?	
...participate fully in meetings?	

(continued)

Do team members...	Yes / No / Sometimes
...welcome the opportunity to take on new tasks delegated by the leader?	
...share decision making as appropriate?	
...have a clear understanding that sharing leadership is an expectation?	

The shared leadership element requires strengthening when one or more of the above questions is rated a "Sometimes" or a "No."

Reflection and Application for Leaders

Increasing the Team's Participation in Decision Making

1. Review the four levels of influence in Figure 7.1.
2. For each level, list recent decisions that have been made at that level in your team.
3. Review the decisions made at levels 1 and 2, and identify any that would have benefited from being made at levels 3 or 4.
4. List the benefits that might have been achieved if the decisions had been made with greater involvement from the team.
5. Reflect on upcoming decisions that need to be made. Identify those that can be made at levels 3 or 4, and begin to develop an action plan for involving the team in these decisions.

Reflection and Application for Everyone

Participating in Shared Leadership

Consider whether you contribute fully to your team.

- Do you see supporting the health of the team as part of your job?
- Do you participate fully in meetings?
- Do you welcome shared leadership opportunities?
- Are there shared leadership opportunities that you would like to have that are not available now? If so, how can you communicate this to your team leader?

Jot down any thoughts on how you might contribute even more fully, not just to your role, but to the team.

8

Shared Learning
Propelling the Team Forward

There is no such thing as the status quo. If growth isn't happening, deterioration is. No matter how collaborative team members may be, the team cannot function at its best unless learning is an ongoing priority.

Each individual learning experience moves the team forward. But learning together and sharing knowledge with one another results in exponential learning, which propels the team farther and faster toward exceptional patient care than could be achieved any other way.

Shared learning is at the heart of a culture focused on quality and performance. The degree to which team members reflect on experiences, share knowledge, and provide feedback to one another in a blame-free, "what can we learn from this" manner, reflects the extent to which the team will be able to fully achieve their quality goal.

In the private sector, when organizations don't make learning—and the application of that learning toward innovation and growth—a priority, the organization goes into decline, losing out to its competitors and suffering financial loss. In the healthcare world, when organizations don't make learning a priority, it is ultimately the patient who suffers.

> "Team learning is vital because teams, not individuals, are the fundamental learning unit in modern organizations. This is where the rubber meets the road; unless teams can learn, the organization cannot learn."
>
> —Peter Senge, *The Fifth Discipline*

In *The Fifth Discipline*, Peter Senge points out that when teams are truly learning, not only are they producing exceptional results for the team, the organization, and, in the case of healthcare, the patient, but the individual team members are also experiencing positive growth more rapidly than they could working independently. Team learning, he emphasizes, is vital because it is largely through teams that organizations achieve their objectives. Development of the whole team, and not just learning within individual professions, is essential to the high-performance healthcare team.[1] *Shared learning* propels the team farther and faster toward exceptional patient care than could be achieved any other way.

So what does *shared learning* look like? It looks like a group of nurses gathered around the nursing station and not just chatting but sharing their patient experiences and asking questions that spark learning. It looks like an obstetrical unit of midwives, nurses and physicians taking 10 minutes to huddle at the beginning of a shift to share any new learning that team members may have gained from the previous shift that might benefit the next. It looks like a team of oncology nurses and physicians in the chemotherapy room discussing a chemo spill, which occurred the day before, to find ways of preventing a spill from occurring again. It looks like an interprofessional team holding a debrief after a procedure and discussing not only what should have been done differently, but also reinforcing what went well. It looks like physicians walking around the floor and speaking with nurses, asking for their opinions and sharing learning and experiences with them. It looks like a team openly reviewing patient-safety incidents at a team meeting for the purpose of finding solutions to prevent the incidents from happening again. It looks like a nurse at a bedside, coaching a student on how to assess a patient experiencing complications after surgery.

It's easy to overlook *shared learning* because its absence is not as easily recognized as the absence or weakness of other elements. It is easier to recognize when the climate element is weak and conflict is strong, or when the cohesiveness element is weak and members put their own needs above the team's. The absence of learning is not as easily noticed. It can drop to the bottom of the list of priorities when other "to-dos" and acts of busyness take over the team; *shared learning* may not even get on the list.

Learning has traditionally been seen as an isolated event rather than an ongoing process. And often it is something that gets relegated to the human resources and educational services departments, and that takes place in a classroom or via e-learning on-line.

If growth isn't happening, deterioration is.

Too often learning opportunities are not recognized or not seen as sufficiently important to be supported. In a discussion on *shared learning*, a nurse lamented the loss of her team's customary meetings: "We used to take the time to have team meetings where we would focus on a specific goal or challenge the team was experiencing so we could work together to achieve or resolve it, or share learning experiences and really tap into each other's knowledge. These meetings were great; it gave us a chance to connect, check in with one another and make sure we were on top of what was happening on the floor that day, week, and month. But since we've grown in size, we've gotten so much busier and we have so many different personalities on the team now that it just doesn't seem to happen."

It is unlikely that management at this nurse's healthcare facility took into consideration the lost learning opportunities when it made the decision to disband team meetings. Or perhaps the meetings were simply allowed to fade away because their importance wasn't recognized.

SHARED-LEARNING PRACTICES

Traditional learning through workshops and e-learning continues to be important. But this alone does not have sufficient impact on the overall effectiveness of a team, especially if the learning is not shared, reinforced, and applied, so that the learning actually "takes" within the team. If a team is to share learning, the team must live the following four behaviours and practices:

1. Voluntarily and readily share knowledge and experience with one another, which includes learning from mistakes.
2. Be open to receiving feedback and providing feedback to one another.
3. Take time to reflect on, and discuss, how to improve care practice, service delivery, and team effectiveness.
4. Approach the discussion of errors in a blame-free, "what can we learn from this" manner.

EVERYDAY LEARNING

> "The best and most cost-effective outcomes for patients and clients are achieved when professionals work together, learn together, engage in the clinical audit of outcomes together and generate innovation to ensure progress in practice and service."[2]
>
> —The National Health Service Management Executive

Learning occurs naturally within the team when it becomes part of the team culture, and recognizing and using learning opportunities becomes part of the daily work process. Learning can occur formally and informally. Formal opportunities for learning include in-service training for the team to update and build new skills, mentoring programs, learning within huddles or short meetings that are dedicated totally to reflecting on how to improve upon service delivery, and learning during debriefs of harm or near-harm events.

Informal learning happens organically when the team culture supports it. It happens when people provide one another with feedback, or ask for feedback; when people share with their colleagues their experiences and learning from a training session or conference; and when people, one-on-one or in an informal group, look for "teachable moments" by using an event, such as a patient fall, to discuss—in an open, non-judgmental manner—how to prevent it from happening again. Learning happens through taking the time to simply ask "What do you think?" and encouraging others to develop critical thinking.

BARRIERS TO *SHARED LEARNING*

Shared Learning Is Not a Priority

Without full commitment from leaders and team members to make *shared learning* a priority, they will not give the necessary time, energy, and commitment, and learning will fall to the bottom of their to-do list—if it even makes the list at all. Without full commitment, learning will be ad hoc and unorganized, resulting in wasted opportunities to prevent errors and improve upon service delivery and team performance. When both the front line and senior leadership fail to embrace learning as a key priority, it is often due to a lack of focus or understanding of the benefits that formal and informal learning opportunities can bring to the team's goal of delivering exceptional care, not to mention the benefits that learning can bring to the well-being and professional development of the staff. Learning will be made a priority when the team and senior leadership address each of the following questions:

- *How does learning from one another and from errors and near misses support our goal (or how does a lack of learning impede our ability to achieve our goal)?*

  Developing a common picture of how learning is directly linked to the team's ability to achieve its goals will help team members to dedicate greater time and energy to the act of learning from one another and from patient-safety incidents.
- *What does shared learning look like in action?*

  Learning is a broad term that can elicit a variety of definitions and examples depending on who you speak to. In order to prioritize learning, the team members must clarify the various ways that learning occurs (or should occur) within their team, both in informal and formal ways. Some learning opportunities, as we have stated previously, occur spontaneously, and others require more formal processes and structures to be incorporated into the team's routine. These more formal processes may include implementing a means of reporting, reviewing, and learning from near misses and errors, implementing interprofessional rounds, or dedicating time within each team meeting to the sharing of ideas to improve the patient experience.
- *Is shared learning a team value?*

  For learning to take root within the team it must be reflected in the daily behaviours of each team member. For some, this will require stepping out of their comfort zone, as it will necessitate committing to practices that may not come naturally. An example of one such practice is being receptive to feedback, and taking time to mentor and encourage critical thinking rather than supplying answers with a knee-jerk response. To support an environment conducive to learning, these changes in behaviour not only require personal commitment, but also the team's commitment to keeping one another accountable. This more readily happens when learning is embraced as a team value.

When *shared learning* is embraced as a key priority and as a living value within the team, the next two barriers, reluctance to ask questions and blame and fear, can be addressed in a more effective manner.

Reluctance to Ask Questions

Questions are the most potent catalyst for learning. Questions that are formulated in someone's mind, but are never asked, are a huge waste. Fear is the common root of reluctance to ask questions, but sensitivity can also be a cause.

On occasion a nurse will shy away from asking newly graduated nurses and nursing students questions that spark learning, such as "What do you think?" or "What prompted you to take that approach?" for fear that the less experienced nurses may think the more seasoned nurses are testing them or finding fault. Learning is stifled when questions are seen as criticism, or when individuals in leadership roles resist asking questions because they don't want others to believe they're being critical.

Limiting beliefs also prevent people from challenging the opinions of others, from asking questions, and from providing feedback to one another. Assumptions and beliefs such as "Nothing is ever going to change, so why bother," "Doctor so-and-so is unapproachable," and "Don't ask questions—it makes you look stupid" block learning opportunities.

There are times when team members will argue that those beliefs are facts. Such a time was pointed out during a discussion with a group of nurses in a nephrology team. When we asked how effectively they believed they worked with the physicians in their department, the nurses shared the impact that more challenging personalities had on their readiness to ask questions. They then expressed how much more difficult it is for the younger nurses, who are new to the team and therefore more easily intimidated. These nurses had learned to simply not ask questions of certain doctors or share opinions with certain doctors, because it was the nurses' belief that these doctors "are who they are, and they will never change."

A similar scenario was described by nursing students and newly graduated nurses, who referred to relationships with their assigned mentors. While some described very positive experiences where they felt free to ask as many questions as they needed to, others reported a more closed environment in which their learning was stifled due to a number of beliefs, including the belief that by asking questions they would be seen as a burden by more experienced nurses, and would appear incompetent. These beliefs stemmed from the behaviour of their mentors, who frequently responded to questions with rolled eyes and sighs, and with comments such as, "Go find the answer yourself," or "You should know that by now."

These are the types of situations that members of a strong team, who have committed to learning together, will tackle by checking their perceptions. If they believe their perceptions are accurate, they will strategize to find ways of developing communication with the seemingly difficult individuals.

Will members be able to capitalize on every learning opportunity if it requires behavioural change on the part of someone else? Perhaps not, but chances are great that the team can make inroads. When someone gives a negative response to questions, they are likely unaware that they are limiting learning. It is important that team members not allow the response of one or two individuals to discourage them from squeezing as much learning as possible from others. Knowledge is power. Imagine the power if all individual knowledge were shared with others.

Leaders can make inroads in creating a culture that embraces learning by practicing the art of asking questions and incorporating simple coaching techniques into everyday conversations. An effective leader turns everyday conversations into learning opportunities—or, "teachable moments"—by adopting a conversation pattern that incorporates questions and sparks critical thinking. Leaders can also make learning a priority by encouraging mentors, nurse managers, nursing coordinators, and other leaders on the front line to create a habit of asking questions of others, and by demonstrating a positive response to those who ask them questions. For a structured approach to incorporating powerful questions into everyday conversations please see Chapter 12: The Leader as Coach.

Fear and Blame

Errors provide critical learning opportunities, but that learning will be stopped in its tracks in an environment where finger pointing, blame avoidance, and defensiveness are the norm. In this type of environment, events that represent exceptional opportunities to learn and improve care practice, service delivery, and patient safety are instead covered up or not talked about. Or, if they are discussed, the intent is to find fault rather than to prevent the event from happening again. In a blame culture, fear of punishment and judgment prevail and self-preservation takes priority over learning in the best interest of the patient and the team.

Much has been written and talked about in healthcare regarding the need to move from a blame culture to a blame-free or just culture. The purpose of reviewing an incident, harm event, or near miss should be to determine the cause from a system's perspective and identify ways of preventing the event from happening again, rather than finding individual fault.

Learning together from errors does not remove the personal accountability essential for individuals and the team to continue to develop and deliver the best care possible. Accountability, however, can only be achieved when teams approach errors and near misses by asking "what can we learn from this?" rather than "who can we blame for this?"

Marilyn Paul, an expert in organizational accountability, states that when organizations move from a culture of blame to one of accountability, they recognize first that "everyone may make mistakes or fall short of commitments," and second that "becoming aware of our own errors or shortfalls, and viewing them as opportunities for learning and growth, enable us to be more successful in the future."[3] This can happen only when individuals trust that when they bring forward an error, near miss, or other learning opportunity, they will not be punished or judged negatively, but acknowledged for being transparent and taking ownership of putting patient safety and the quality of care first, and for helping themselves and the team to improve and learn together.

In 2010, the American Federal Aviation Administration (FAA) announced that the number of reported incidents rose 81 per cent since 2007, from 1,040 reported incidents in 2007 to 1,887 reported incidents in 2010.

Upon first glance, this revelation might startle the average person and create concern; however, Diane Spitaliere, manager of media relations for the FAA, stated that passengers should not be alarmed by the increase in errors. Part of the increase, she explained, was due to better reporting methods implemented in 2008. The new method protects controllers from punishment for errors they voluntarily report. Since the non-punitive culture of error reporting went into effect, the FAA says it has received about 250 reports a week.[4]

"The FAA's mission is to keep air travelers safe," Spitaliere said. "Over the past several years, the FAA has transitioned to a non-punitive error-reporting system at its air traffic facilities. This cultural change in safety reporting has produced a wealth of information to help the FAA identify potential risks in the system and take swift action to address them."[5]

A culture of blame and fear is dangerous. Not only does it erode morale, motivation, and commitment, it also stifles learning and can prevent a team and organization from uncovering problematic systems issues that could impact the safety of patients and staff alike. The Institute of Medicine reported that "the biggest challenge to moving toward a safer health system is changing the culture from one of blaming individuals for errors to one in which errors are treated not as personal failures, but as opportunities to improve the system and prevent harm."[6]

Blame and fear prevails in a team when

- There is a lack of trust.
- There is consistent unresolved conflict.
- People question the intent of others.
- Errors and near misses are met with punishment and judgment rather than being regarded as opportunities to learn and find solutions.
- Individuals regularly find fault with others.
- There is a feeling of "everyone for himself or herself" as opposed to "we're all in this together."
- There is finger pointing; focusing on the person rather than on behaviours, systems, and processes is the norm.
- Leaders do not actively encourage and promote the importance of reporting near misses and errors.

- Leaders do not effectively provide constructive and positive feedback on a regular basis.

LEARNING THROUGH ERRORS

> "An organisation's ability to learn from failure is measured by how it deals with both large and small failures, not just by how it handles major, highly visible crises or accidents."[7]
>
> —A. C. Edmonson

The importance of creating blame-free cultures is, for the most part, recognized in healthcare facilities, and some hospitals are taking significant action to ensure that reporting and learning from errors becomes the norm. In 2012, the McGill University Health Centre (MUHC) and the Jewish General Hospital in Montreal, Quebec, began posting data on their websites concerning medical incidents and accidents. Practices like these are creating the transparency that is so essential to being in sync with requirements for thriving in the twenty-first century. But perhaps even more importantly, when hospitals publicly acknowledge errors, they model what they have been asking their staff to do. The reporting of errors is an important first step to an essential *shared-learning* opportunity.

Patricia Lefebvre, coordinator of the MUHC patient safety, quality, and performance department, and her team are making inroads to increasing staff reporting of events. Lefebvre emphasizes the critical role of reporting events in improving safety and quality. Reporting has increased at MUHC, but encouraging reporting continues to be a priority for the team. They ensure that once an event is reported, the event debriefing leads to learning. Importantly, the team debrief is led by a trained facilitator who is able to create a safe and open environment, and ensure that a productive, focused discussion takes place so that optimal learning can occur. The team is subsequently kept posted on the outcomes of any recommendations that emerge from the debrief. These practices encourage continued engagement in identifying and learning from events.

MUHC might be described as a hotbed for learning. Learning starts with the hospital's values. Having leadership as a value is not unique, but MUHC takes leadership a step further by referring to learning when describing their leadership values in their mission statement: "We develop, use and disseminate continuously new knowledge and expertise that can benefit patients locally and globally."

It is well known that MUHC's aim of learning through research has led to medical advances. But the same commitment to learning is seen across the hospital.

In nursing, the team is leading the Transforming Care at the Bedside initiative in which staff members learn from one another and their patients, and put processes in place that improve quality, efficiency, and the patient and family experience, as well as strengthen interprofessional practice. Front-line process-improvement teams made up of interprofessional staff and patients identify areas for improvement on the unit, and conduct simple tests of change with pre- and post-measurements. They use a structured approach, "Rapid Cycle Improvement," which increases learning and its effective application.

In its first year, the initiative produced several significant improvements, including redesigning a chemotherapy room, decreasing the time at start by 57 per cent, and introducing a quiet zone for medication documentation, which resulted in a 50 per cent reduction in interruptions and a 60 per cent reduction in errors.

Effective teams that employ *shared learning* and are fanatically focused on creating a total quality experience for patients have unlimited possibilities.

Powerful energy is released when learning is sparked.

"The learning process is something you can incite, literally incite, like a riot." Although the word "riot" might have a negative connotation, this quote from author Audre Lorde is one of our favourites because it suggests so well the energy released when powerful learning is effectively sparked.

It becomes self-propelling once people are engaged. Learning means growing, and growing brings new vigour to individuals and teams. Looking for and experiencing learning opportunities can be an exciting adventure.

REFLECTION AND APPLICATION

Signs That the Shared Learning Element Is Strong

Leaders can conduct a quick check of their team's *shared learning* with the following assessment. Assign a response of Yes, No, or Sometimes to each of the following questions.

In my team...	**Yes / No / Sometimes**
...are questions as common as statements?	
...do members look for opportunities to share their learning and knowledge?	
...is there a blame-free environment in which members are encouraged to report and discuss errors and near misses?	
...do members dialogue with one another to find innovative solutions to problems?	
...is sharing knowledge encouraged?	
...are members brought together regularly in huddles, briefings, or debriefings to share learning or to problem solve?	

The *shared learning* element requires strengthening when one or more of the above questions is rated a "Sometimes" or a "No."

Reflection and Application for Leaders

1. Learning as a Priority

It is up to leaders to engender a learning environment. Check the following questions to see if there is an area of opportunity for you.

Take a few minutes to reflect on how you encourage learning experiences in your team.

(continued)

- Do you make learning part of the team conversation?
- Do you make time on the team meeting agenda to invite questions, concerns, and issues relating to patient safety, the quality of care, or team performance?
- Do you encourage an open-door policy where team members know they can always approach you with questions and concerns?
- Do you respond to questions, issues, and errors in a manner that positively reinforces the act of speaking up rather than assigning blame?
- Do you approach errors in a "what can we learn from this" manner?
- Do you take time to coach your team members?

For any question you answered with a "No" or a "Sometimes," create a list of things you can do to incorporate the practice on a regular basis. For tips on how to incorporate coaching into everyday conversations, see Chapter 12: The Leader as Coach.

2. Incorporating Everyday Learning Opportunities

For each of the following *shared learning* scenarios, determine how often the scenario occurs within your team using the following scale: 1: Never, 2: Rarely, 3: Sometimes, 4: Frequently, 5: Always.

- Team members share their patient experiences and ask questions of one another that spark learning.
- Huddles are held at the beginning of each shift to share any new learning that team members may have gained from the previous shift that might benefit the next.
- Interprofessional debriefs are held to discuss what went well and what could have been done differently with a patient case/procedure.
- Physicians walk the floor and speak with nurses and other professionals, asking their opinions and sharing learning with them.
- The team reviews patient-safety incidents together for the purpose of finding solutions to prevent them from happening again.

For any scenario rated a 3 or less, identify what you and your team can do to begin to implement the practice.

(*continued*)

Reflection and Application for Everyone

1. Reflect on *Shared Learning*

Reflect on each of the following quotations and ask yourself if there is a personal meaning in it for you. If so, is there an action you and/or the team would benefit from your taking?

Note that quotations can also be used in team meetings to trigger reflective discussion.

"Every person in this life has something to teach me—and as soon as I accept that, I open myself to truly listening."—Catherine Doucette

"Where all think alike, no one thinks very much."—Walter Lippmann

"You aren't learning anything when you are talking."—Lyndon B. Johnson

"It is what we think we know already that often prevents us from learning." —Claude Bernard

2. Renew Your Curiosity

Can you remember the curiosity with which you entered the healthcare profession? It is likely that everything was new; everything was exciting; everything triggered a question. That feeling of curiosity is often dulled by routine or simply by striving to survive in what can be a very stressful environment.

Learning becomes automatic when we are curious. Ask yourself, "How can I renew my own curiosity? How can I help my team do the same?"

Part II

Making It Happen: Achieving Improved Team Performance

9

The Team Development Process

The most important requirement to effectively developing a high-performance patient-focused team is commitment. Commitment has to be felt at a level deep enough to ensure follow-through. It is easy to be intellectually committed. Plenty has been written about how effective teamwork leads to better patient care. Anyone who has worked in or led a group of individuals knows from experience the enormous difference that effective teamwork makes to both the staff and patient experience.

If the benefits are so obvious, why then isn't every healthcare unit implementing a team development process? Perceived obstacles prevent people's commitment from moving from their head to their heart, where passion lives. Without passionate commitment, the way things are done is seldom changed. The reasons are many. Leaders may be intimidated by the prospect of developing a team. Perhaps there are team members whose behaviour is so entrenched that the leader feels there is no way to influence change. Others may believe they just don't have time, or there is no use because the organization's culture is not team oriented. Fear caused by lack of knowledge creates doubts that stall action. People ask: *Where do we start? How do we go about it? How do we know that any intervention actually makes a difference and isn't a short-term blip before things go back to where they were? How can we change when the rest of the hospital is not fully embracing teamwork?*

As people begin to recognize the importance of teams and their direct link to quality patient care, every leader across a healthcare organization will be required to learn how to build effective teams. Our book is designed to help leaders take their team forward. Once a leader grasps how to develop a team and, through learning the team development steps, can envision the difference team development makes to patient care and the staff experience, the leader's commitment becomes firm. Once leaders begin to see the results, the commitment becomes passion.

THE TEAM DEVELOPMENT PROCESS

One-time team events or interventions may create short-term change and benefits, but all too often old practices and behaviours soon resurface. These ingrained practices and behaviours, then, were never actually altered—they just went underground for a bit. The real danger of one-off interventions that do not provide lasting results is that some staff members will believe that they have proof that these sessions don't work, and so will be less receptive to the next try. Basically, one-off interventions can give team development a bad name.

We are not suggesting that an event for teams can't have benefits such as energizing the group, providing an opportunity to productively discuss issues or problem solve, or providing an opportunity for team members to better get to know one another. However, if the purpose is to support the development of an effective, patient-focused team, then these events need to be part of something larger and ongoing.

When team development makes a lasting difference, it is because it has become an ongoing and critical team practice. This is a practice for which not only human resources or the leader, but all team members take ownership. Getting to that point may feel like an onerous task, but once the process is in place and team members see, and very importantly *feel*, the results, growing the team becomes a seamless part of "the way we do things around here." At that point, when the fabric of the team transforms, and you have achieved a cultural change.

The team development process is a structured one with easy-to-follow steps as shown in Figure 9.1.

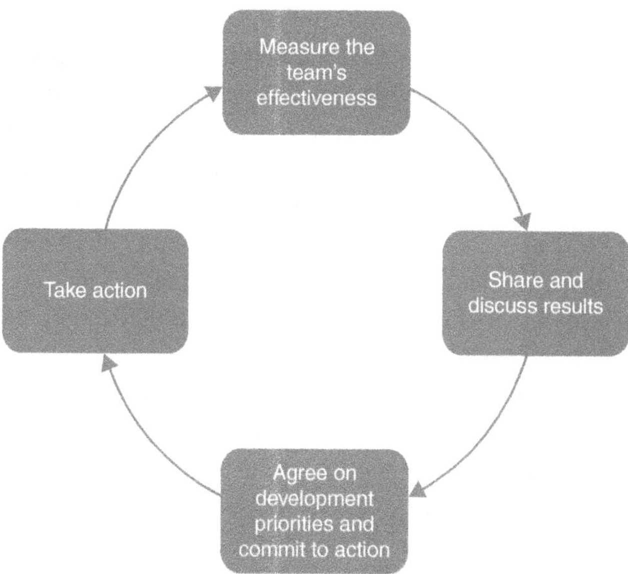

Figure 9.1: The Team Development Process

MEASURE THE TEAM'S EFFECTIVENESS

Using an Assessment

Assessing the team's effectiveness has the obvious benefit of providing data about the team's strengths and growth opportunities. It provides a benchmark from which to build, and it clarifies and/or confirms the areas that the team must focus on in order to move toward becoming a high-performance team that optimally supports both patients and members. In order for a team to develop, it must clearly understand the improvements required to increase team effectiveness. Team members usually have ideas about how their team could improve. Few, however, have specific knowledge about what is required for high-performance teamwork. Therefore, even when a team is consciously making an effort to improve, it could overlook critical aspects that may be blocking team performance. The assessment results also provide an excellent framework for structured discussion, which is essential to a team development process.

Assessment results provide the leader with much valuable information in addition to assessing team strengths and growth opportunities. For some team leaders, the results will confirm that the leader's estimation of his or her team members is correct, and that the leader has been accurately tuned in to his or her team. Other leaders may find the results surprising. The assessment may reveal that the team is more effective than the leader thought. Or, on the other side of the coin, the assessment may identify weaknesses that the leader overlooked. When the latter is the case, the leader may feel stressed that the team's practices and behaviours are seen as "worse" than they had expected. In actuality, this is a gift, an amazing opportunity for leaders to acquire information that they can use to excel in their role and lead their teams forward.

Importantly, the results identify the priority areas that most immediately require attention. The responses also indicate to what extent team members have similar views about the team and how it works.

A common and highly valuable—but less obvious—benefit is that the team members will be more engaged in the process. By completing the assessment, members come to own the results. Rather than the leader, human resources, or even a pocket of members determining the need for team development, the team itself determines or confirms the need, as well as the development priorities. When introduced effectively, the team development process becomes something done "by us" rather than "to us."

An assessment also increases the commitment level, because people more readily pay attention to what is measured. What is measured tends to gain more respect than what is not. It is more likely to be viewed as something that deserves attention.

A final benefit is education. By completing an assessment and being involved in subsequent discussions of the results, members come to understand the essential elements of a high-performance team and the behaviours and practices that are essential to their own performance as a team member.

What to Assess?

The seven elements of high-performance teams that we have described in this book provide a framework for assessing team performance. They can educate the team about the key elements that are non-negotiable if team members are to demonstrate high-performance teamwork.

Comprehensive team assessments can be purchased or developed by the internal human resources group. If a budget is not available, the mini assessments we provide for each element, at the end of chapters 2 to 8, can be used to effectively launch and structure a team development process.

Introducing the Team Assessment and Development Process

Achieving buy-in from team members is in great part determined by the leader's ability to effectively communicate the purpose of the assessment and the team development process that will follow. The following is the key information to be shared before inviting members to complete an assessment.

1. The Purpose of the Team Assessment and Development Process

Teams at all levels of fitness, from those that are functioning very well but want to be even better, to those that are facing some team-effectiveness challenges, use a team development process to tap into the best of themselves. At the heart of the team development process is a team assessment, the purpose of which is to provide each team member with the opportunity to share their perspectives on how their team is functioning. Once completed by the team, the results of the assessment will provide insight into the team's key strengths and essential growth opportunities, and provide focus and structure for the team's ongoing development.

In some teams and organizations there is a fear of assessments, because members believe that assessments are used to find fault and to punish, rather than for the purpose of learning and growth. In these environments, it is especially important to clearly communicate that the purpose of the assessment is to help the team to work together more effectively, so that the staff can have a more positive daily experience and thus provide their patients with the best possible care. Clarify that the assessment is a vehicle to help identify and celebrate strengths, and to more accurately target the areas requiring attention, so that the team can take action—together—to fully tap the team's potential.

2. The Importance of Being Open and Honest

The assessment gives team members the opportunity to voice their opinions and to communicate what they perceive to be the team's strengths and weaknesses. Ask that team members read each question carefully and take the time to reflect before choosing their response. The more open people are, the more helpful the results will be in effecting real change within the team. Individual responses will remain confidential and anonymous.

It is important for individuals to feel safe in providing open and honest feedback. This is especially the case for teams in which tensions are high and/or the culture leans toward one of fear and blame rather than one of openness and trust. Taking steps to ensure confidentiality and anonymity will improve the response rate and will result in more honest and accurate feedback. It is important to communicate to the team that only cumulative team data, not individual responses, will be shared with the team.

3. Next Steps: How the Assessment Data Will Be Used

Healthcare professionals and teams are often inundated with assessments, from employee satisfaction and engagement surveys to assessments mandated by accreditation bodies. Oftentimes surveys are conducted and individuals never receive follow-up information regarding the outcomes of the surveys and how the results will be used. This causes survey fatigue and skepticism regarding the benefits of surveys, and creates a belief in many that surveys are a waste of time. Clearly communicating how the results will be used and how and when the results will be shared (and living up to these commitments) will help leaders begin to combat any skepticism at the onset. It is helpful to communicate the following:

- When the assessment will be administered, and when and how it needs to be returned
- Approximately how much time is required to complete the assessment
- When and how the results will be shared with the team (see the Share and Discuss the Results section below for more detail)
- How the results will be used (see the Share and Discuss the Results section below for more detail)

SHARE AND DISCUSS THE RESULTS

The results make the greatest impact when shared soon after the survey has been completed. Team members will be curious about them, and immediate follow-up demonstrates that the initiative is a priority. As indicated above, sharing the results in a timely manner communicates the message that the results will in fact be used to help propel the team forward.

Taking time to reflect on the results before sharing them with team members is essential to a successful discussion of the results. Think about how they will be presented, and how the discussion will be facilitated. The sharing and discussion of the results is the first development step that the team takes as a group, and as with many things in life, the first impression can strongly influence things to come.

Whether it is the leader or an individual from outside of the team who facilitates the meeting, the leader's demeanour and responses during the session strongly influence the tone, team members' openness during the discussion, and the team's subsequent level of engagement in the development process. Whether they leave with a "things will never change" attitude or with great hope for an even better team experience depends greatly on the degree to which the leader projects a personal commitment to the process and to supporting team members in making any required change. It is critical that the leader conveys a genuine willingness to be the first to make any personal change required to ensure the team's success. This will help enable team members to more readily receive input and make personal change.

CAUTION

If team issues are sensitive and/or the leader's behaviour is perceived to contribute to team dysfunction, it is recommended that a facilitator from outside the team leads this and future team development sessions until the team resolves its key issues and is sufficiently developed to continue the process by themselves.

Depending on time available, one meeting may not allow for full discussion of key results. And, depending on the size of the team, several meetings might be required in order to involve all team members.

AGREE ON DEVELOPMENT PRIORITIES AND COMMIT TO ACTION

In this step the team agrees on the areas it must focus on in order to best strengthen the team. Using an assessment makes reaching an agreement easier because the assessment results highlight the areas that the whole team believes require improvement. Therefore, priorities for the most part have already been agreed upon.

The *commitments to action* (CTAs) emerge from the team's closer examination of its growth opportunities. For example, if the team identifies that the open communication element requires strengthening, the question for the team is, "What do we have to do to strengthen this element?" The recommendations generated and agreed upon become the team's set of CTAs. (For guidance on how to achieve consensus on the commitments to action, refer to Chapter 11: Facilitation: The Skill that Determines the Success of the Process.)

TAKE ACTION

What happens after the meeting or between meetings is equally important. Teams that best follow through on their CTAs find ways to reinforce them and build upon them on a regular basis. This can happen at a start-of-shift huddle or during regular team meetings. The New Patient Referral Team at Hamilton Health Sciences' Juravinski Cancer Centre is an example of a team that demonstrated true commitment and follow-through throughout their team development process. Their process began with the use of the Healthcare Team Fitness Assessment, which incorporates the seven elements of a high-performance healthcare team, and resulted in the team coming together regularly to continue their development.

In the initial stages the team developed CTAs for addressing key areas for improvement, for keeping each other accountable to them, and for maintaining their team development momentum. The team made working together effectively as much of a priority as their day-to-day responsibilities. Below is a sample of their CTAs and the template they used to stay on track. Each team member kept a copy, and it was updated after each team development meeting.

COMMITMENTS TO ACTION

New Patient Referral Team

Week 1: Discussion of Assessment Results

The following represent the CTAs developed after sharing and discussing the assessment results:

Climate

- Accept apologies
- Allow team members space
- Maintain humour, allow for free expression
- Maintain a non-judgmental environment

Team Members' Contribution

- Fair contribution from all when DST/Phys/Mgr needs help
- Ask for help when needed
  - Co-worker
  - Manager

Following the initial meeting, in which the team shared and discussed their assessment results and identified the above commitments to action, the team committed to meeting on a regular basis to participate in team development exercises ranging in length from 15 minutes to one hour, in order to address areas the team identified as impeding their performance. (Team development exercises are provided in Part III: The Tools to Make It Happen.)

The following represents the commitments to action developed after participating in each exercise.

COMMITMENTS TO ACTION

Week 2: Managing Assumptions

ASSUMPTION: Coming to a conclusion not based on fact.

Commitment to Action

1. If I am uncertain about a co-worker's behaviour or comments, I will ask for clarification privately, if appropriate.
2. I will remind or question myself:
   - "Am I making an assumption?"
   - "Do I know this for a fact?"

Team Commitment

The New Patient Referral Team agreed to "pause" each morning for 10 minutes to review their team-building commitments. This is also an opportunity for team members to discuss any work-related topics/news.

Week 3: Preventing Future Conflict

Commitments to Action

1. Communication: I will be mindful of how I approach a colleague, of my tone of voice, of my non-verbal behaviour, and of my choice of words.
2. Differing Response to Change: I will support and help those who are struggling with change.
3. Assumptions: If I am uncertain about a co-worker's behaviour or comments, I will ask for clarification privately, if appropriate.
4. I will remind or question myself:
   - "Am I making an assumption?"
   - "Do I know this for a fact?"

Week 4: Response to Conflict

Commitments to Action

1. Be calm, take time out to lower emotional charge before trying to resolve the conflict.
2. When a co-worker is tense, be careful not to make assumptions.
3. Put personal feelings aside. Do not take differences of opinion personally.
4. Respectfully advocate for my beliefs.

KEEPING UP THE MOMENTUM

The New Patient Referral Team used their CTAs at team meetings to check on their progress. Effectively using the CTAs kept the team focused on the areas they identified as requiring the most improvement in order to move forward as a high-functioning team.

When teams get off track and don't follow through, it is often because the goals and commitments they have made are lost among a sea of daily tasks. If the leader and team commit to carving out "sacred" time, which is set aside solely for team development, it will ensure that the team's momentum won't be lost. This does not require a great deal of time.

The team development time might be 15 minutes at the beginning of regular team meetings, or huddles dedicated to checking in and reviewing CTAs.

A simple but powerful way to increase follow-through on commitments and ensure the team takes action to improve performance is to ask team members what they believe they need to do in order to keep each other accountable for their commitments. Team members might agree to remind one another if they slip, or agree to a buddy system where buddies provide one another with feedback.

CAUTION

This technique of holding one another accountable is not always possible at the early stages if the climate and open communication elements are weak.
As the team develops these elements, team members become more comfortable with and effective in providing each other with support through feedback.

TIP

For larger teams it is helpful to create a *champion team*, a small group of team members responsible for ensuring that team development is kept at the top of everyone's mind and helping the team follow through on its CTAs. The champion team becomes responsible for scheduling team development meetings, for conducting short but purposeful team development exercises at the beginning of team meetings (some can be found at

(*continued*)

www.healthcareteamperformance.com), and for keeping the team on top of their CTAs. It is helpful if the champion team reflects the makeup of the team, one individual representing each profession, and it is essential that each member commits to modelling positive team behaviours. The development of a champion team helps to communicate to members that team

REASSESS

Too often we see teams make great strides by assessing themselves and using the results to bring about real change, only to never assess themselves again. These teams miss the opportunity to not only affirm and celebrate any progress they have made, but also to reinforce the change so that it sticks over the long term. The reassessment is the proof of the pudding: it provides teams with verification that their efforts to change really do make a difference, and therefore provides the motivation that many need to maintain the process and prevent the team from slipping back into old habits.

The reassessment also provides helpful data that can be correlated by the team, senior management, or HR with other data such as employee satisfaction, patient satisfaction, and other performance indicators to demonstrate that team performance truly does impact the staff experience and the quality of care.

Teams committed to team development conduct an assessment on average twice a year, and for teams in crisis we recommend they complete the assessment more frequently so that team development becomes a priority, and necessary behaviour change occurs more quickly.

TIP

Reassessment is a time for recognition and celebration of the progress the team has made. Taking time to not only share the results but also to have the team share their success stories and what they have observed about the team's progress creates a burst of energy that continues to move the team forward.

AN ONGOING PROCESS

Once the team development process has been established, it is an ongoing process for which the team must take responsibility. The greatest danger is the leader and team resting on their laurels and feeling that they have "made it."

High-performance teams' secret to success is the regular monitoring of their team effectiveness, which ensures they catch any slips before they become weaknesses that can put their performance at risk. The creation of a champion team, as mentioned earlier, is a powerful way to ensure that team development is ongoing and not an intervention with a start and end date.

Team development has no expiry date. Team fitness, like physical fitness, requires assessment and commitment to improve targeted weak spots. Commitment to the fitness process results in team flexibility, well-being, and dramatically increased performance, which leads to better patient care and a healthier work environment for all.

A TEAM DEVELOPMENT QUICK START: CLARIFYING EXPECTATIONS

Should the team and/or leader determine for whatever reason that a complete team development process, as described above, is not feasible, the team can benefit greatly from taking time to clarify the expectations that each member has of the team, their teammates, and their leader.

Like individuals, teams have very distinct personalities, and become dispirited when expectations are not met. Clarifying expectations can greatly enhance a team's ability to work together effectively. When teams lament their lack of spirit, morale, or zest, members usually have a list of unfulfilled expectations. Some of the unfulfilled expectations are big issues, and are often, to a great degree, uncontrollable. For example, the team has no control over limited resources. But the items that cause the most grief and eat away at team morale are the little things. Often team members walk around with their own secret wish list and assume that somehow those expectations will be fulfilled.

"I shouldn't have to ask for help when I'm overloaded. I expect others to be sensitive enough to help when necessary," explained a frustrated team member to her colleagues in a session held to clarify team expectations.

What is a perfectly obvious and reasonable expectation to one person may not occur to someone else, or may even seem entirely unreasonable.

After this team member clarified her need for others to offer assistance proactively, her colleagues spoke up and clarified their own behaviours. One team member explained that when she has offered to help other people in the past, she has been accused of assuming that others were incapable of doing it on their own. As a result, she decided that instead of opening herself to criticism, she would wait until someone asked for her help. Another team member responded, "You always seem like you have everything under control, so I figured you would ask for help if you need it, like I do. I assume everyone is as busy as I am and probably don't notice when I'm overwhelmed. But I know if I ask for help I'll get it. Now that I know you'd prefer the assistance to be offered, I'll do so when I can."

It became evident that a culture of "everyone for his/herself" had evolved due to different expectations around giving and receiving assistance. Once these expectations were clarified and assumptions were challenged, the team committed to both asking for help when needed and offering to help others when capable of doing so.

In another instance, a *professional practice leader* (PPL), who was responsible for facilitating the team meetings, described how frustrated she was with team members showing up late to meetings or leaving the meetings early. She explained that it made her feel that team members didn't care about the team and the information being shared, and that she found it disrespectful given the time she committed to the team meetings. The team members who had been arriving late or leaving early clarified that their behaviour was due to last-minute issues relating to patients, who they believed took priority over the meeting, and that their late arrival or early departure from meetings was no indication of their support for the PPL or the team.

The discussion led to an agreement that they would let the PPL know ahead of time whenever possible if they would be leaving early or arriving late. This may appear to be a seemingly simple clarification, but it is one that went a long way in alleviating the misperception that certain members of the team were behaving disrespectfully—a perception that, on clarification, was found to have been held by several members of the team, and not just the PPL.

High-performing teams have clear expectations. Their expectations are usually made clear by having team members come together to list and examine them. When teams function effectively, expectations are as follows:

- Articulated
- Clarified
- Given a reality test; and, if realistic
- Agreed to

Clarifying expectations can be a very quick working tonic for teams that are not fulfilling their potential. The types of issues identified by examining expectations will, of course, differ depending on the team's place within the organization, its mandate, and its level of development. The benefits, however, are consistent.

Clarifying expectations

- Allows team members an opportunity to address unfulfilled expectations without personalizing them (pet peeves are positively and productively aired)
- Allows for open discussion of new issues
- Results in increased understanding (may explain why expectations aren't met, how perceptions differ, and the ways in which certain expectations are unrealistic)
- Establishes the underlying expectation that open communication will be the norm

The expectations that the team agrees to in effect become ground rules. A group of individuals can't be expected to play as a team without agreed-upon rules. We refer to these ground rules as *team agreements.* A process for clarifying expectations and developing team agreements is provided in Part III: Tools to Make It Happen.

Developing Team Agreements

Team agreements stem from team members' expectations of one another, and define the behaviours and practices the team identifies as essential to the team's effectiveness. The following reflects a set of team agreements developed by a rehabilitation team.

In order to be an even better team, we agree to do the following:

- Listen to and respect one another's opinions.
- Provide regular, positive feedback to each other (i.e., recognize achievements).
- Respect each other and our individual roles in the larger group (i.e., no role is less than or more than any other role).
- Respect our individuality and the different ways each person approaches work.
- Make administrative decisions only when all relevant staff have given input.
- Not to let concerns/frustrations about the team or individuals fester—we will address those that we feel need to be addressed.
- Provide a solution when communicating an issue to be resolved.

In order for team agreements to work, they must be used. Developing them at a team meeting and never referring to them again will not result in positive behaviour change. A member of a group, that was not functioning well, once complained that clarifying expectations and developing team agreements were a waste of time. Her team had spent a whole day developing a long list, and nothing had changed. When we asked when her group had last looked at its list, she shrugged and said, "Well, the day we developed it."

The purpose of developing team agreements is to clarify expectations and to facilitate a change in individual and team behaviour for the better. This can only happen when team agreements are reviewed, updated regularly, and kept at the top of everyone's mind. Many teams keep their agreements posted for everyone to see, and the most effective teams take time regularly to assess themselves against the agreements to ensure that the team is living up to them. Once an agreement has become a team norm, in that the behaviour is now being practiced consistently, the agreement can be removed and replaced with a new one. Team agreements identify the behaviours and practices that require improvement within a team. Once improvement has been achieved, it is important to recognize the success, acknowledge it, and replace the agreement with a new one that reflects another behaviour and practice essential to becoming an even better team.

Clarifying expectations and developing team agreements is a good spot check and maintenance tool for high-performance teams, and an effective re-energizer for those experiencing lethargy.

10

The Leadership Balancing Act

The key to being effective is balance. This holds true for an organization as a whole and for a team, leader, or front-line worker. We have become even more aware of balance recently because many of today's issues are framed within this concept. We strive for balance in our lifestyle, our career and home life, our diet, and our caretaking of the environment. Balance is equally required for us to function effectively at work, whether that entails leading a healthcare team or caring for a patient.

Workplace balance requires managing two sets of behaviours and practices, which may be seen as polarities; however, each is required in order to function effectively. At one end of the continuum are task-oriented behaviours, and at the other end are process-oriented behaviours. Being task oriented is a heads-down, "let's get down to business" approach to working. It includes providing structure and direction, paying attention to detail, taking a logical approach to decision making and problem solving, and making firm decisions. To a great extent, the focus is on *what* needs to be done.

Process orientation at the other end of the continuum is a heads-up, "let's look around and gather information" approach to working. It includes focusing on the big picture, sharing information, seeking input, and making people the priority. The main focus is on *how* things need to be done. The art of team leadership is being able to move with ease from one end of the continuum to the other at precisely the right moment.

Although some people are naturally balanced in their practices and behaviours, and are able to easily move across the continuum between task- and process-oriented behaviours as needed, most people have a natural preference for one or the other. Both *task* and *process* are essential

Table 10.1: Task/Process Modes of Operating

Task	Process
Independent: Is most comfortable working alone.	**Interactive:** Is most comfortable when working with others.
Detached: Deals with things objectively.	**Attached:** Displays emotion and sensitivity.
Inward Looking: Focuses on details.	**Outward Looking:** Focuses on the bigger picture.
Logical: Uses facts and logic.	**Intuitive:** Uses creativity and intuition.
Convergent: Brings things to closure.	**Divergent:** Opens up discussion and looks for alternatives.

to effective leadership and teamwork, and one is not more important than the other. Table 10.1 describes the preferences associated with each mode. It is when a leader shows a strong preference for one end of the continuum, and automatically operates from that end, that he or she is at a disadvantage.

Leaders who operate primarily from the task end of the continuum, for example, will demonstrate effectiveness in getting things done and making decisions. Leaders at this end of the continuum, however, will be at a disadvantage in certain ways. For example, they will not consistently demonstrate process-oriented behaviours that are essential to achieving consensus and ensuring that "people factors" are taken into consideration. When the process side is weak, the leader may struggle to create an inspired and committed team. However, the task side is responsible for efficiency, without which a leader cannot gain the respect required to be an inspirational role model.

Once you realize where your personal imbalances lie, you can begin to develop new practices and behaviours that will allow you to increase your effectiveness.

THE INCREASED NEED FOR BALANCE

In addition to one's natural preference for task or process behaviours, there are several factors that may nudge healthcare leaders toward demonstrating task behaviours. The healthcare profession and the disciplines within it are trained to be task oriented, with logical problem-solving and decision-making processes and attention to detail. The very nature of a fast-paced job, with numerous critical responsibilities and large spans of control can result in leaders adopting a heads-down mode of working, choosing unilateral decision making, and providing solutions and giving directions rather than engaging team members.

At one time managers could get away with limited attention to the process side. Authority got the job done well enough, expectations were not as high, and the world was not as transparent. The link between patient-focused teams and quality care had not been made. Change came slowly. This allowed the task-oriented healthcare facility and its people to function well enough in the task mode with their heads down, sharing minimal information, working in silos, and telling rather than asking.

Today such behaviour reflects weakness on the process side, which most commonly creates an imbalance in the healthcare leader's approach. If the process side is weak, the leader is not sufficiently in tune with his or her team to recognize early on if there is an issue, and so may not address it quickly enough. When leaders are weak on the process side, they do not create strong interpersonal connections with team members and can therefore appear to be uncaring. That does not mean that they don't care. They perhaps do care but don't make the caring visible. They use objectivity and logic at the expense of sensitivity and intuition, which are also required to bring out the best in people.

Some leaders are by nature very high on the process side—at the expense of the task side. A leader needs a healthy task side in order to perform the management portion of his or her role. Without sufficient task orientation, the leader misses details and makes errors. His or her communication may be too broad and not sufficiently to the point. The leader may not always be able to make logical and sometimes difficult decisions if sensitivity overrides objectivity.

If one's task/process preference is too far to the task side, the result can be rigid, authoritarian management; if one's preference is too far to the process side, the outcome can be limp leadership that results in compromise and appeasement rather than purposeful—but sometimes challenging—decision making.

Leaders who are able to achieve balance are flexible, responsive, and effective. These leaders are facilitative in style—they create the situation in which things happen, rather than forcing things to happen. A balanced healthcare leader looks for opportunities to grow and empower people, collaborate, and build his or her team. In an urgent situation, these leaders tell; in a non-urgent situation, they ask. Perhaps they ask, "What do you think is the best approach?" or "How can we resolve this?" Even in situations where directing or telling is necessary, they maintain a facilitative attitude and approach. A balanced leader gives direction without intimidating, embarrassing, or disempowering people. In any environment, a leader must assess when being facilitative is not the answer and giving specific direction and making quick decisions is critical. Facilitative leadership results in getting the best from a group of people by reshaping a group into a team.

The following is a brief description of each of the *task/process balance* modes. The degree to which the descriptions apply to an individual depends on the strength of his or her preference for a particular mode. If the individual is fairly balanced in his or her preference, descriptors from both sides will apply. In the Reflection and Application section of this chapter, you are provided with a tool to assess your task/process preference so that you can identify both your strengths and your opportunities for improvement.

Independent/Interactive

Individuals who show a strong preference for the *independent mode* will work best on their own. A brainstorming event is not the best venue for them to develop ideas; they need quiet to think and reflect. They often do not think of the importance of communicating certain information that others might expect to receive. They are content to work on their own, not needing the stimulation of others. In order to re-energize, they need time alone.

Individuals who show a strong preference for the *interactive mode* work best as part of a group. They need company and think best when sharing thinking processes with others. They re-energize by being with people. Communication is important to them, and at times they may communicate more than people around them would prefer.

Leaders with a strong preference for the interactive mode tend to communicate openly and invite others to share decision making and give input and feedback. They are also quick to give recognition and feedback to others. However, as always, there can be too much of a good thing, and too much participation, meeting, and talking can be unproductive if not managed and designed to produce outcomes.

A Note to Leaders with a Preference for the Independent Mode

Leaders with a strong preference for the independent mode are self-reliant and are comfortable solving problems and making decisions on their own; however, this preference brings downsides when it relates to leading teams effectively. Unless they are aware of how working in the independent dimension impacts their effectiveness and make adjustments, it is likely that in addition to not readily sharing information, they will not bring their team members together often enough, and will not readily share decisions, invite input or feedback, or provide sufficient feedback or positive reinforcement.

Transparency has become an important issue throughout healthcare and at every level of an organization. We have worked with leaders who were perceived as non-transparent, even manipulative, because they did not share information that others believed was their right to have, or that others thought was important to successfully fulfilling their roles. Although, on occasion, this perception was true, we found that more often these individuals were highly independent and didn't think of sharing information.

Detached/Attached

Individuals who show a strong preference for the *detached mode* are able to stand back from issues and examine them objectively. They value factual information and may discount softer evidence. They don't readily show emotion and don't take things personally.

As leaders, they may be well positioned to deal with team issues and conflicts and to do so fairly. In healthcare, objectivity and the ability to detach from emotion can be critical to the well-being of the staff and to their ability to objectively communicate with and treat their patients. The lack of expressed emotion, however, can result in a cool approach to the people they lead and care for, which can be interpreted as lack of caring and sensitivity.

Individuals who show a strong preference for the *attached mode* become emotionally invested in issues. On the one hand, they may have difficulty being objective, but, on the other, the emotional investment can translate into enthusiasm for an initiative and eagerness to contribute. These leaders are highly compassionate and demonstrate that they care for their team members, and embrace and champion issues they believe in. They respond to issues with sensitivity. However, a high preference for this mode may result in leaders emotionally taking sides in issues and having difficulty making hard decisions where people are concerned. Leaders who operate mostly from this mode are likely to take things personally and be more concerned about how they are perceived by others, which makes making the tough decisions even more difficult. Leaders who operate predominantly from the attached mode may look for compromise and try to make everyone happy rather than find the best decision for the organization and team.

Inward Looking/Outward Looking

Individuals who have a strong preference for the *inward mode* work well with detail but can get so caught up in it that they miss the bigger picture. They need clear goals and objectives, and work best within a structured environment.

Leaders with this preference may spend too much time with their heads down and miss important clues or information from the teams they lead. Their strong focus on detail in their communication can fail to motivate members who are more outward looking and need a broader perspective—members who need to have things linked to a bigger picture.

Individuals who have a strong preference for the *outward mode* are tuned in to the bigger picture, are good at seeing the ramifications of a particular action, and may speak in broad terms or generalities (preferring not to work with detail).

Leaders who are highly outward looking may miss important details and fail to provide their team members with comprehensive knowledge and information necessary for the team to perform at its best. They may assume understanding. They understand and build the important links between their team and others across the organization. They keep mission, vision, and goals in front of their team.

Logical/Intuitive

Individuals who have a strong preference for the *logical mode* like the world to make sense. They like to approach things in a step-by-step manner. They need to understand the "why," and have difficulty fully supporting a change that, to them, is not logical and therefore not the best way to do things. Their decisions are based on facts and figures. It can be difficult for them to see another's point of view or to let go of their own. They can play a devil's advocate role in challenging ideas. They ensure people have their feet on the ground.

Leaders with a strong logical preference can have difficulty rallying their team to implement a change that the leaders don't understand or with which they don't agree. Their need for understanding might make them behave in a way that the team perceives as negative, making the leaders poor models for the team members they lead.

At the same time, their step-by-step style might build a good organizational foundation for the team, and their tendency to probe for better understanding can enlighten everyone.

Individuals who have a strong preference for the *intuitive mode* are tuned in to ideas and the people around them, and they get a quick sense of what will work and what won't. They like to explore possibilities. They are open to others' ideas and to trying new approaches. They present creative solutions, but these solutions may not be confirmed by facts at hand. They work best in a self-directed, unstructured environment.

Leaders with a preference for the intuitive mode are confident decision makers. They are able to create energy and fun with their liberal thinking. They easily pick up on and build on others' ideas. They have a strong aptitude to lead and facilitate groups because they can quickly read the members' responses and the group dynamics. The downside is that their preference for a freewheeling approach can result in too little structure, and the team's performance may then suffer.

Convergent/Divergent

Individuals who have a strong preference for the *convergent mode* hold firmly to their strong opinions. They are quick to make decisions and reluctant to change them. These leaders become impatient with discussions that they see as "wheel spinning." They are frequently the ones that bring decision making to closure. They are more likely to tell than to take the time to ask or involve others.

When the preference for the convergent mode is strong, individuals may have difficulty as leaders because their behaviours echo traditional top-down management. The manager makes a decision and tells people what to do and how to do it. Leaders with these tendencies find that learning about participative leadership and diligence in self-management allows them to lead effectively.

Individuals who have a strong preference for the *divergent mode* are open to others' views and like to gather as much information as possible before making decisions. They take a facilitative approach to dealing with people. They probe and ask rather than tell. They look for compromise when opinions differ.

These natural tendencies can bode well for an individual's success in leadership; however, leaning too far to the divergent side can result in wheel spinning and too much compromise, both of which affect the productivity and morale of a group.

* * *

One of the most important steps in self-development is to know oneself. In order for leaders to hone their leadership skills, it is important for them to understand which leadership behaviours they are most comfortable with and come most naturally to them, while at the same time identifying those behaviours that don't necessarily come naturally but are important to leading a successful team.

BALANCING THE TEAM'S TASK/PROCESS PREFERENCE

Leaders have to be cognizant of not only their own balance, but also that of the teams they lead. Like individuals, teams have a distinct task/process preference. Their makeup might be well balanced, resulting in an ability to move easily and effectively back and forth between task and process. Most teams, however, do not have that balance naturally. A team is likely to have a predominance of either task-oriented or process-oriented members. As with individuals, if the task orientation is high, the team is likely to be very efficient, but may not always solve problems creatively or make the best decisions. They are likely to produce outcomes that do not have the buy-in of all team members.

On the surface, process-oriented teams appear to be made for a world of change. They are flexible, open to new ideas, like to talk things through, and look for creative solutions. In spite of these powerful abilities, they seldom fulfill their potential because they miss details and struggle to bring things to closure.

Being cognizant of a team's task/process balance assists its members in making the adjustments required to allow the members to work together to produce superior outcomes. With this knowledge the group can better share the responsibility of creating an effective team process. By knowing the group's makeup, the leader is better attuned to the team's tendencies. He or she can more easily tell when the team is out of balance and is likely to be led astray.

REFLECTION AND APPLICATION

The Leader's Task/Process Balance

A. Understanding Your Personal Balance

For each scale provided below, mark where you believe you most often sit on the task/process continuum.

Below each scale, make a note of your strengths and most positive behaviours and practices. If you do not consistently rest close to the centre of the scale, note any behaviours you think are under-represented and any you think are over-represented. Here's an example of a leader of a long-term care unit. This self-assessment can be downloaded at www.healthcareteamperformance.com.

Independent ______________________________X________ Interactive

Strengths:

- Holds regular meetings
- Interacts regularly with staff

(continued)

Over-demonstrated behaviours and practices:

- May talk too much in meetings, and shut others out as a result
- May interact to the point of slipping on administration duties
- Interacts too much with some members and not enough with others

Under-demonstrated behaviours and practices:

- Does not take enough planning time
- Depends too much on others for decision making

* * *

Independent ______________________________ Interactive

Strengths:

Over-demonstrated behaviours and practices:

Under-demonstrated behaviours and practices:

Attached ______________________________ Detached

Strengths:

Over-demonstrated behaviours and practices:

(continued)

Under-demonstrated behaviours and practices:

Inward Looking ______________________________ Outward Looking

Strengths:

Over-demonstrated behaviours and practices:

Under-demonstrated behaviours and practices:

Logical ______________________________ Intuitive

Strengths:

Over-demonstrated behaviours and practices:

Under-demonstrated behaviours and practices:

(*continued*)

Convergent ____ Divergent

Strengths:

Over-demonstrated behaviours and practices:

Under-demonstrated behaviours and practices:

B. Readjusting Your Balance

If you find you are consistently much closer to one end of the pole than the other, a readjustment is likely in order so that you can capitalize on your strengths. For some it means learning new skills, and for others it requires that they push themselves out of their comfort zone. But for most it means small tweaks and reminders that they need to behave in a manner that they are already familiar with, but that they may forget on occasion, slipping into the mode that comes most easily.

The following is an easy way to begin to make the adjustment. However, it requires consistency.

Revisit Part A and consider your own task/process balance for each dimension. Then select a behaviour or practice that would move you closer to the centre of the scale, and would positively impact the health and effectiveness of your team. Make a personal commitment to consistently adopt that behaviour.

Take five minutes of quiet time daily to reflect on how well you are doing—to pat yourself on the back when you are succeeding, and to reprimand yourself if you aren't. It takes vigilance to change behaviours.

(*continued*)

Once those behaviours have become habit, add another, and then another to your personal balancing act, until you are performing at your best as a team leader.

It is likely you have found that there are some behaviours that you have learned to demonstrate positively most of the time, even though they are not within your naturally preferred mode. But when under stress, you may revert to less effective behaviours. If you know ahead of time that you have to deal with a stressful situation, it can be helpful to remind yourself of the behaviour you need to demonstrate to be effective, and to visualize yourself in the situation responding with the appropriate balance. The more you consciously practice the new preferred behaviour, the less effect stress will have on your behaviour of choice.

Athletes improve their performance by visualizing the perfect scenario. Leaders can do the same.

11

Facilitation

The Skill that Determines the Success of the Process

The success of the team development process will be in great part determined by the leader's ability to effectively facilitate open dialogue that leads to quality decisions that are fully supported by the team. Much of the team's formal development will occur during team meetings, in which team members come together to clarify expectations and identify and commit to specific actions and new behaviours. If the team leader lacks effective facilitation skills, the meetings will fall flat and fail to produce decisions and action items that are fully supported by the team. At best, the team will pay lip service to the commitments, and, at worst, the meeting could result in greater conflict and a lack of trust in the team development process. The good news is that facilitation skills can be learned. The processes, tools, and skills shared in this chapter provide a structured and practical approach to leading productive meetings, whether these are team development meetings, or any meetings in which the participation of the attendees is required, where decisions are made, and where consensus is important.

Those who facilitate team development most effectively have the fine task/process balance described in the previous chapter. The facilitator must be not only focused on the task at hand, including agenda items, discussion content, and time, but must also be focused on group dynamics, including individuals' participation, body language, and any unspoken messages. It is this balanced attention that produces productive outcomes.

THE FACILITATOR'S POWER TOOLS

Highly effective team development sessions flow with such ease and flexibility that to the participant or casual observer they appear quite unstructured. Underlying that free-flowing process is a well-planned structure executed with intuitive flexibility. Exceptional facilitators lead meetings with ease, effortlessly bringing people together, encouraging the sharing of opinions and ideas, and managing difficult behaviours in a manner that creates cohesion. Upon first glance it appears that these individuals are naturally gifted facilitators, and for some this is the case. But, more often, exceptional facilitators work hard to prepare with knowledge and a set of tools, processes, and skills that allow them to create the perception of ease and natural ability.

What differentiates exceptional facilitators from all the rest is the set of tools at their disposal that allows them to effectively manage the group process. In this chapter we share five learning bites[1] that include the knowledge and tools most essential to facilitating a team development meeting:

1. The Requirements for an Effective Meeting
2. Meeting Agreements
3. Team Decision Making: Achieving Consensus
4. Generating Dialogue and Participation
5. Managing Conflict

Facilitation Learning Bite 1: The Requirements for an Effective Meeting

There are six basic requirements that can determine the success of the facilitator and the meeting:

1. Clarify objectives
2. Stay on track (topic and time)
3. Ensure full participation
4. Clarify understanding
5. Ensure commitments to action
6. Recap

Clarify Objectives

It is the facilitator's responsibility to clarify the objectives of the meeting. This basic step is often missed, and is one of the biggest culprits when it comes to discussions getting off track. Meetings often start with the facilitator jumping right into the first agenda item instead of clarifying the purpose of the meeting. The objective describes what the group wants to achieve. The most common complaints about meetings is that they get off track—discussions take on a life of their own and have little to do with the topic at hand. This occurs because the objective is either forgotten or never defined to begin with. Taking two minutes at the beginning of the meeting to clarify exactly what the group is to achieve by the end of the meeting will help keep the discussion on track and on time.

The meeting objective can then itself become a meeting-management tool. When the discussion gets off track, the facilitator can pause the discussion and ask the group, "Is discussing the issue we are having with patient flow going to lead us to our objective of identifying how to improve our bedside reporting process?" Team members can then more easily agree to stay focused on the objective at hand. When the objective is known and reinforced throughout the meeting there is less chance that unrelated topic will be brought up.

Stay on Track (Topic and Time)

In healthcare, time is a rare commodity, and the time spent in meetings must be well used and outcomes highly productive. Staying on track and on time may seem like a small responsibility; however, there is nothing more frustrating than coming to the end of a meeting feeling as though you've accomplished nothing and have wasted your time. When meetings veer off topic for too long and time is wasted, it is often the result of one of the following:

- Objective was unclear or forgotten
- Too many items on the agenda
- Insufficient time allotted to important topics
- Inability of the facilitator to balance his or her attention to task and process

It is the role of the facilitator to ensure that the participants don't veer off topic and lose track of time. A well-developed agenda with clearly defined objectives wssill help the facilitator to keep on track, and will help to ensure each agenda item is essential to the topic at hand.

Keeping the meeting on track requires that the facilitator pay close attention to ensuring a balance between task and process. Task-oriented individuals have a greater tendency to push the discussion along too quickly, wanting to get through all of the agenda items on time; speed, however, often comes at the expense of quality. In contrast, a process-oriented individual may linger too long on a topic, allow too much discussion and idea generation, and may not be able to get to all of the items essential to the objective.

Balancing attention to task and process requires that the facilitator keep a close eye on the dialogue, recognizing when it is appropriate to bring the discussion to a close and move on to the next item, and recognizing when more discussion is necessary. Staying on track requires facilitators to be flexible. They should recognize when it is appropriate to get off track, and make a conscious decision with the group to do so. Being off track becomes a problem when the group is wandering and the facilitator doesn't realize it, or doesn't do anything about it.

Ensure Full Participation

Different people have different participation styles. Some prefer to think quietly and absorb the information shared prior to speaking up, and others are far more vocal, eagerly jumping into the conversation. Full participation does not mean that everyone gets equal airtime, as this does not suit everyone's personality. It does mean, however, that everyone must have an equal opportunity to participate, and that all participants contribute to the process. A good general guideline for full participation is that *if participants have an idea they express it; if participants have a concern they share it.* If individuals have something important to say, they say it in the meeting, not over coffee later. We share a number of tools to support full participation throughout this chapter.

Clarify Understanding

Do not assume that everyone understands what has been said. Clarify understanding of important points and points of view, especially on sensitive issues. In Chapter 2 and Chapter 4 we discuss the dangers associated with assumptions, and how assumptions create blocks to communication and impede the development of trust. It is the facilitator's responsibility to help challenge assumptions and clarify understanding by

- Regularly recapping key points and confirming the group's understanding
- Asking questions in order to probe more deeply into an important topic so that everyone is on the same page
- Asking whether members have any questions, or if anything requires greater clarification or discussion, rather than assuming everyone understands and is on the same page (it is key to remember that silence does not equal agreement and understanding)

Ensure Commitments to Action

Although discussing strengths and growth opportunities can in itself be therapeutic for some teams, performance improvement requires that the discussion culminate in team commitments to action (CTAs). This requires consensus on the CTAs, and clear next steps as appropriate, such as who, what, and when.

Recap

Like clarifying objectives, recapping is often a step that is missed during meetings, even though it provides a number of benefits to the team development and meeting process. Taking a couple of minutes at the end of a meeting to recap what has been agreed to ensures that everyone leaves the meeting with the same understanding. It increases the likelihood of follow-through on commitments that are made. It helps ensure that the group leaves the meeting with a sense of accomplishment.

* * *

While it is ultimately the responsibility of the facilitator to ensure that each of the above requirements is fulfilled, taking time with the team to review the criteria for a successful meeting will support the development of their meeting skills. This time can also be used to make it clear to the team that an effective meeting is everyone's responsibility. The team can also use these six requirements to assess their effectiveness at the end of a meeting. Table 11.1 provides a template for assessing meeting effectiveness (it can also be downloaded from our website at www.healthcareteamperformance.com).

Table 11.1: The Meeting-Effectiveness Barometer
Consider the effectiveness of your meeting by rating each of the following requirements on a scale of 1 to 4.

	Not Well			**Very Well**
How well did the team:	**1**	**2**	**3**	**4**
Clarify objectives?				
Stay on track (topic and time)?				
Ensure full participation?				
Clarify understanding (of all points discussed)?				
Ensure commitment to action?				
Recap outcomes?				

Facilitation Learning Bite 2: Meeting Agreements

A positive team development process is dependent to a great extent on the quality of the dialogue among team members. When discussing team concerns, participants must be able to raise potentially sensitive issues and give and receive feedback. Although the facilitator creates an environment in which these things can happen, team members must take ownership of the way they communicate.

Before a discussion begins, ideally team members identify the behaviours required for a positive process, and agree to demonstrate those behaviours. These are called meeting agreements, and they describe positive behaviours that the team identifies as essential to working together effectively during regular team meetings and/or team development sessions. For example, an agreement might be, "We agree to listen openly to all ideas." These agreements are not generalities or platitudes. They are based on previous meeting experiences, and will reflect team behaviours that, in the past, did not productively move the meeting forward.

A set of meeting agreements helps to clarify what team members need from one another in order to be open, and clarifies the requirements for a "safe" environment. It also gives members permission to be open. By developing and referring to the agreements as needed throughout the workshop, the facilitator helps create a positive process. Here is an example of a set of meeting agreements:

We agree

- That all feedback be given with a positive intent
- To listen to each other's points of view without interrupting
- To participate in the meeting by sharing ideas and opinions
- To approach every discussion in a blame-free, "what can we learn from this" manner

It is important to involve everyone in developing the agreements so that they are not perceived as rules imposed upon the team, but rather shared commitments made in an open and comfortable setting. The process is a simple one. The facilitator asks the group to respond to the following question: "What do you/we need from one another in order to have an open, positive, and productive meeting?" The facilitator then captures the responses on a flip chart so that the agreements are visible throughout the meeting. The facilitator can use the agreements in the same way that he or she employs clarified objectives: as a meeting-management tool that can be referred to throughout the meeting as needed.

Facilitation Learning Bite 3: Team Decision Making: Achieving Consensus

Ultimately the group's effectiveness is reflected in the quality of the decisions it makes. In conducting a team development session in which a variety of opinions and ideas will be presented, the facilitator needs to be armed with tools to structure the discussion and help ensure the team reaches an outcome that is fully supported by all team members. Most teams see consensus as the ideal decision-making method. At the same time, many find consensus difficult to achieve, and, as a result, some leaders shy away from a consensus process, assuming that it will take far too much time and that it carries the risk of never achieving consensus at all.

The benefits of a consensus process, which will help drive the decision successfully forward, include the following:

- Enthusiastic buy-in
- Better decisions, which result from dialogue that is essential to the consensus-reaching process
- Thorough understanding of issues, which leads to more effective implementation of the decision

Consensus is required when one or more of the following apply:

- The team is addressing an important issue.
- The team members are directly affected by the decision.
- The team members' understanding and behaviour can affect whether the decision works (buy-in is required).

All of the above apply to team development in which the team members work together to determine new practices and behaviours that will improve team effectiveness.

One of the greatest impediments to consensus is misunderstanding or different understandings of what consensus means. Expectations of consensus range from "a decision with which there is wholehearted, 100 per cent agreement" to "a decision that everyone can live with." The first can sometimes be achieved, but it is often an unrealistic expectation; the second does not aim high enough. "Living with it" doesn't suggest the energy or enthusiasm that will be required to make the decision work. The following definition most effectively guides consensus-reaching processes:

Consensus is agreement to support the decision 100 per cent.

Supporting a decision is different from agreeing with the decision. A nurse or physician may not agree 100 per cent with the Electronic Medical Record system the organization adopted, but if the decision-making process is properly managed, they can agree to *support* the decision 100 per cent.

When leading a team toward consensus, it is important that the team understands what *consensus* means and what the term *support* means. In order for a team member to demonstrate support, he or she must

- Speak positively about the decision and take ownership of it outside of the meeting (for example, saying, "we decided" not "they decided")
- Do whatever is required to make the decision work

In team development, team members must reach consensus on their commitments to action. If there is true consensus they will show their support by doing whatever is required to ensure they live up to their commitments and by fully owning them. The commitments to action must truly be *our* commitments to action.

Team members' support often depends more on how they perceive the process than on whether they like the decision. In order for team members to fully support a decision, they must know that their ideas and concerns have been heard, and must understand (not necessarily agree with) the rationale behind the decision.

The following provides a step-by-step approach to more easily achieving consensus:

1. **Clarify the definition of consensus:** When sharing and discussing the definition of consensus, ensure that members understand what supporting a decision looks like in action. Each member must understand what is expected of them when they are asked to support a decision.
2. **Agree on a back-up plan:** If the team is unable to achieve consensus, how will the decision be made? Back-up plans include the following:

- Passing the decision on to the leader or person(s) most directly involved in making the decision work
- Deciding by majority vote

If all members agree to support whatever decision is made via a back-up plan, in essence you have still achieved consensus.

3. **Use tools to structure the process:** The Generating and Organizing Ideas Technique, presented in the following section, enables individuals to share ideas and gain greater understanding of a topic or decision. Structure is the key to success.
4. **Recap and confirm:** Once a decision has been made, confirm that a consensus has been reached, remind members that they are expected to support the decision, and reiterate what support entails.

   In order to test for true consensus, particularly on sensitive and important issues, it is important that the facilitator, having first reminded the group of the expectations attached to the word *support*, checks with each member. Ask specifically, addressing members by name. For example, "Sarah, do you support this?"

Tips for Consensus

Often a few individuals enthusiastically support an idea and others, who perhaps were earlier opponents, are now quiet. It can appear that these individuals are now in agreement. However, they may simply have been worn down, or, for some other reason, have chosen not to register their disagreement. Others, by their nature, may not vocally support the decision. A few enthusiastic positive responses to the question, "Have we reached an agreement?" does not a consensus make. Ensure that enough time is scheduled to thoroughly check for consensus.

On one hand, it is important not to rush consensus. On the other hand, groups often spend much more time in discussion than is necessary to reach consensus. Once you sense that all ideas have been heard and considered, and members have focused on one or two options, ask whether the group is at a point where it can reach consensus. You might say, "Are we at the point at which everyone can support one of these ideas?" Very often the answer is yes, and a great deal of time is saved. If the answer is no, repeat the question periodically to both move the group along and to check its progress.

Facilitation Learning Bite 4: Generating Dialogue and Participation

At the heart of a successful team development process are dialogue and participation, both of which can present challenges for the facilitator. When we lead facilitation training workshops, some of the most common questions we are asked relate to dialogue and participation.

- How can I get everyone involved?
- How can I prevent an individual in a more senior position from inhibiting others' participation?
- How can I increase the quality of input and ideas?
- How can I prevent a few vocal people from driving the process and most strongly influencing the outcome?
- How can I keep the discussion focused?

We have one answer to each of the above questions: structure. With the right structure in place even the most timid of individuals will participate, and even the most enthusiastic of individuals will be contained in a manner that doesn't stifle their enthusiasm. The following structured approach is called the *Generating and Organizing Ideas Technique*, and when it's used effectively, it produces quality outcomes that are fully supported by the group.

The Generating and Organizing Ideas Technique (GOIT) (see below) was inspired by the nominal group technique (NGT), a classic facilitation tool. The NGT was developed in the late 1960s by André Delbecq and Andrew Van de Ven as a program-planning method. It has since become a tool that no meeting facilitator leaves home without. It is referred to in a number of the team development exercises presented in this book. The GOIT is a means to

- Increase participation and therefore the number of ideas generated
- Protect ideas and participants by preventing judgmental responses
- Provide a structure that helps keep the group on track and allows it to achieve its objective in an efficient manner

THE GENERATING AND ORGANIZING IDEAS TECHNIQUE

The Generating and Organizing Ideas Technique consists of the following six steps:

1. Clarification of the problem, objective, or topic
2. Silent generation of ideas
3. Round robin feedback of ideas
4. Clarification and discussion of each recorded idea
5. Reaching agreement
6. Commitments to action

This is a useful technique that can help to

- Develop workshop, team, or meeting agreements.
- Identify opportunities for improving team performance.
- Develop commitments to action.
- Brainstorm ideas.

This technique is effective for

- Generating a lot of ideas
- Keeping discussion on track
- Ensuring participation from every team member
- Achieving outcomes
- Achieving consensus

The Generating and Organizing Ideas Technique offers you several options for collecting and sharing the ideas that are generated. Members may share their ideas verbally, anonymously on a piece of paper to be read by the facilitator, or on a sticky note that members will not share verbally but stick on a flip chart or board.

Decide in advance on the mode of participation that will work best for the particular meeting. If a number of team members are highly uncomfortable speaking out in the group, or if the issue is a sensitive one—which could inhibit participation—you may decide to have ideas put forward anonymously. This method of participation should not be used routinely and should not be necessary once a team begins to develop. It is important that everyone is comfortable participating, but equally important that open participation, in which individuals contribute verbally and take ownership of their ideas, becomes the norm. If the team is developed enough to share ideas openly, have all members put forward their ideas themselves.

The third option is a compromise between the other two. Members write their ideas on a sticky note and stick it to the board. They take ownership for the idea by posting it, but don't have to share it verbally and are not asked to put their name on it.

The Six Steps of the Generating and Organizing Ideas Technique

Step 1: Clarification of the Problem, Objective, or Topic

As we outlined in Learning Bite 1: The Requirements for an Effective Meeting, taking time to confirm understanding of what the group is setting out to accomplish is an essential first step. Without it, members may be working at cross purposes or move off track.

Step 2: Silent Generation of Ideas

In this step, team members are asked to quietly consider the issue to be discussed and to jot down their ideas. Ask that these few minutes (five minutes is usually sufficient) be silent time. Participants can collect their thoughts and so increase the quality of their contribution as well as the likelihood that they will volunteer their ideas. If participants are inexperienced in the participation process, this brief preparation time can greatly increase their comfort level. In addition, many more original ideas will be generated. When a discussion is unstructured, the first people to put forth an idea will influence the thinking of other members and can limit original thinking. (See Table 11.2 for more options for generating ideas.)

This step has many benefits:

- The facilitator sends the message that everyone is expected to contribute.
- Everyone quickly gets into the process and begins to think about the topic.
- Team members who tend to work best independently and quietly have the opportunity to collect their ideas in a manner that works well for them.
- Each member is doing original thinking, not influenced by others' thoughts.
- The number of suggestions generated is greatly increased.

Table 11.2: Options for Generating Ideas

Option	Method	Next Step	Benefits
Silent Generation of Ideas	Members write their ideas on a notepad.	Round robin sharing of ideas.	• Increases participation • Creates an opportunity for equal participation • Increases the volume of ideas • Allows for more carefully considered contributions
Anonymous Generation of Ideas	Members write their ideas on a piece of paper, which is given to the facilitator.	The facilitator shares the ideas.	• Allows members to share ideas when a sensitive issue might otherwise limit participation (should be used rarely, as members should feel free to express their ideas openly in most situations)
Building a Wall of Ideas	Blank sheets of flip chart paper are posted around the room. Each member chooses a sheet and writes as many ideas as possible.	The facilitator assists the group in identifying commonalities and combining the ideas into one list.	• Moving around is energizing • Members have thinking time • Members have the opportunity to contribute all of their ideas • Creates a large volume of ideas
Sticky Ideas	Members are given large coloured sticky notes. They are asked to write their ideas on them and post them under the topic heading on a board or wall.	The facilitator assists the group in identifying commonalities and combining the ideas into one list.	• Moving around and the visual effect of the sticky notes are energizing • Large volume of ideas

(*continued*)

Option	Method	Next Step	Benefits
Pass the Envelope	Each member writes an idea on a piece of paper and puts it in an envelope. Each envelope is passed to another team member, who writes an additional idea that is triggered by the idea in the envelope. They write it on a piece of paper and add it to the envelope. The process continues, with each member examining all of the ideas in the envelopes they receive until each member has contributed to each envelope.	Ideas are sorted and compiled in a list (note: takes time).	• Large volume of ideas • Members build on one another's ideas • Encourages creative thinking

Step 3: Round Robin Feedback of Ideas

Record ideas as they are shared so that they are visible to the group. Begin with one idea per person and go around the group. Suggest that people start with the idea or point they feel most strongly about. If time permits, continue until all ideas have been heard. Discourage discussion at this stage. Judgmental remarks can cause members to hold back their comments and lessen the effectiveness of the process. Discussion at this point can also lead to a too-early focus on one idea and/or a premature decision.

Step 4: Clarification and Discussion of Each Recorded Idea

Ensure that everyone has the same understanding of each point. During this step, invite team members to build on and meld ideas. Be cautious in combining ideas, however. It is important to check with participants to ensure they are indeed expressing the same or similar points. Combining ideas too hastily can cause the loss of important ones.

> **TIP**
>
> Establish an agreed-upon length of time for discussion based on the number of ideas generated.

Step 5: Reaching Agreement

At this stage, if the list of ideas requires prioritizing or shortening, some group decision making is required. It is important to facilitate agreement on how the group will prioritize the ideas or select the "best" ideas. This could be as simple as having the team members vote for their top choices, or could include developing a list of decision-making criteria that will clearly define what the decision will be based on. Decision-making criteria might include, for example, any combination of the following:

- Positive impact on the patient
- Improves staff productivity
- Improves staff satisfaction
- Low cost
- Easy to implement

Step 6: Commitments to Action

This is the "where do we go from here" step, with specific commitments regarding who will do what, when. Ensure that everyone agrees to the next steps and captures them as specifically as possible.

Facilitation Learning Bite 5: Managing Conflict

Differences of opinion in group processes, when well facilitated, take the group discussion and the decisions that come out of it to a higher level. Effective leaders and facilitators encourage different points of view. This not only helps move the discussion toward better decisions, but also demonstrates the importance of hearing each others' views, and communicates that each individual has a right to express his or her own opinion, as long as it is presented respectfully. When a group avoids disagreement, there is an increased risk of "group think." Groups whose members tend to quickly agree may appear efficient and collaborative, but they may actually be generating mediocre decisions or worse as they are not challenging one another's ideas.

When to intervene, when to let a discussion based on differing points of view run its course, how to manage conflict when it arises, and, very importantly, how to prevent conflict from occurring at all are pieces of knowledge essential to the facilitation of a successful meeting.

Determining When to Intervene

One of the many decisions a facilitator must make is whether to intervene when differences of opinion arise. Are members engaged in a high-spirited but ultimately healthy debate, or is the interaction dysfunctional? The following provide clues as to whether the discussion is healthy or impeding the group's ability to reach its objectives:

- Are team members attacking one another rather than the issue?
- Are some members uncomfortable with the nature of the discussion?
- Are good ideas or important perspectives not being heard because of the level of emotion?
- Are people not really listening to one another?
- Is the group spinning its wheels? Are members stuck on a heated issue that is preventing them from moving ahead?

An alternative way of determining whether to intervene is simply by asking the group, "The discussion is becoming quite heated. Is this a productive approach to addressing the issue, or do we need to approach it differently?"

Caution: On one hand, if the facilitator is more highly task oriented and more highly detached than attached, he or she may miss important cues that indicate it is time to intervene and take a different approach. On the other hand, he or she may want to move things along too quickly, not recognizing the benefit of disagreement.

A heated debate often involves only a few of the members. That discussion can distract the facilitator from staying in tune with those not engaged in the exchange. Everyone's verbal and non-verbal responses can send important signals to the facilitator. Signals from those not participating could be discomfort or loss of interest, and could warn the facilitator that their commitment to the process may be waning.

Preventing Conflict

Conflict arises most readily when the meeting discussion is a free-for-all, rather than a structured process. Conflict can be prevented by using the tools previously presented in this chapter, which are recapped below:

1. Clarify the meeting objectives so that members are on the same page and know what they are working toward.
2. Develop and use meeting agreements. The key word here is *use.* Meeting agreements must become part of the process and used throughout the meeting as reminders of the positive behaviours that must be demonstrated in order to create a positive experience.

> **TIP**
>
> When developing meeting agreements, ask team members to identify an agreement that describes how they would like to deal with conflict should it arise.

3. Use a structured approach to decision making and brainstorming, such as the Generating and Organizing Ideas Technique.
4. Check for understanding of the points of view presented. Conflict often arises because of misunderstanding. When emotion is at play, one's

hearing can be distorted. Paraphrase the key points: "Let's recap what is being said to ensure that we all have the same understanding."

5. Be assertive. Remember that you are the person who is ultimately responsible for the effectiveness of the process. Don't hesitate to intervene if you think the group may be heading for conflict.

Sources of Conflict

In preparing to manage conflict, it is helpful to understand the most common causes of group conflict.

Different Values

Values are shaped by many factors, including profession, culture, background, and lifestyle. In interprofessional healthcare teams, differing values are often at the root of conflict.

Different Agendas or Priorities

Individuals from different professions or areas within an organization are likely to have different priorities that come into play. When this is the case, it is important to remind the group of the common priority—achieving quality patient care, for example—as a means to find common ground.

Different Work Styles

Different work styles can lead to conflict. Consider these opposites: detail oriented and big-picture oriented; individuals who like to bring things to close quickly and those who like to open up the discussion and mull things over. The opposites in each pair can approach aspects of a group process very differently, sometimes leading to frustration and often conflict. The group can benefit from the differences if the differences are acknowledged and discussed, and if the group recognizes how they can make the most of the strengths each style brings to the process.

Miscommunication

Miscommunication may result from misunderstanding a message, from assumptions being made about the non-verbalized intent behind the message, or even from the sender's body language.

Strategies for Managing Conflict

The facilitator can adopt one of the following practices to help manage conflict situations.

Set the Conflict Aside

If there is a strong difference of opinion that is impeding the group process, but the issue is not directly related to the group's objective, ask the group to set the difference aside. You might say, "It appears that you are not going to reach an agreement on this point. My sense is that it is not necessary to agree on this to meet our objective. Would you agree?" Assuming the group agrees with this suggestion, continue by saying, "I'm going to ask that you set that discussion aside and refocus on our objective for this meeting."

Revisit Meeting Agreements

In the event of conflict, it is likely that at least one of the original agreements has been broken during the conflict. Stop the discussion and ask the group whether they have been adhering to the agreements. Often forcing members to simply recognize that they have not lived up to their agreements will result in members taking ownership of their behaviour and managing it more effectively themselves.

If team members are demonstrating negative behaviour that is causing conflict that had not been addressed by the agreements, ask the group whether anything needs to be added to the set of agreements. If the group does not recognize the negative behaviour, share your observation. For example, "I'm noticing that the discussion is focusing on placing blame rather than finding a solution. Can we add an agreement that states, 'We agree to focus on finding a solution rather than finding individual fault'?"

Clarify Understanding

Ensure that participants understand each other's points of view by inviting one person to recap his or her idea or perspective. Share your understanding of what the individual said or, better still, invite a member who is in conflict with this position to give his or her understanding of what has just been said. Check for confirmation from the individual who owns the perspective.

Invite the other party to clarify his or her point of view and repeat the above step. If there are more than two perspectives, continue until they have all been recapped.

Once the points have been clarified, it is not unusual to discover that the perspectives are actually very similar.

Invite Members to Suggest a Resolution

The conflict may not simply be the result of misunderstanding and emotion; there may be substantive differences. Clarify these points of view and diffuse the emotion, and then invite the members to suggest a resolution.

Be Self-Aware

The facilitator's behaviour and tone strongly influence the course of a conflict situation. The facilitator must

- Remain detached from the emotion of the conflict
- Intervene assertively but positively when needed
- Not appear to take sides

Having a natural task/process balance, as we discussed in the previous chapter, is a huge advantage in facilitation. But as described in each of the five Learning Bites, providing structure and having tools at the ready are the keys to an effective group process.

TIP

We have provided a great deal of information in this chapter. If you are relatively new to the role of facilitator, take one idea or practice from each Learning Bite and, once you are comfortable using them, add more.

12

The Leader as Coach

"Coaching is . . . helping another person reach higher effectiveness by creating a dialogue that leads to awareness and action."

—Anne Loehr and Brian Emerson, *A Manager's Guide to Coaching* (2008)

In Chapter 6: The Sum of the Parts: Team Members' Contribution, we explained that with synergy, the whole is greater than the sum of its parts. However, we emphasized that although synergy should be an aim of team development, we cannot ignore the strength of each of the parts. Leaders can quickly and effectively achieve a higher level of teamwork by devoting time to coaching individual team members in parallel with developing the team as a whole. Unfortunately, excuses like "I don't have time to be a coach" or "I don't know how to coach!" can be common responses to this suggestion.

Coaching is one of the most powerful tools a leader can use to tap the best of their team members and to propel the team forward, and yet it is a responsibility that many shy away from due to preconceived notions about what "coaching" really is. It is often thought that, in order to coach, leaders must block off hours every week to meet with staff, and that they possess a hard-to-define and equally hard-to-grasp skill. Happily, coaching is not a difficult skill to develop or to use. Coaching is simply about having engaging conversations and asking powerful questions.

In order to keep development alive and well within the team, the leader must model positive team behaviours and support others in doing the same. When using coaching techniques, the leader is doing both of these. In the simplest terms, coaching involves asking questions that spark an individual's ability to tap into his or her own critical thinking abilities, skills, experiences, and opinions. When it comes to developing and empowering others, the coach who takes the time to ask before telling—or, preferably, advising—will produce greater results.

"On the job" or "on the run" is probably the best description of how coaching is likely to happen in a healthcare environment. This is the alternative to a regular half-hour sit-down, although, ideally, those are also built into the schedule. It is more likely that coaching will happen on the floor during regular conversations between leaders and their staff. The key is to identify "coaching moments" and to have a simple approach to structuring the conversation so that coaching can happen spontaneously.

GETTING STARTED

Coaching is fully successful only when the individual being coached is receptive. When people expect to be coached, and see it as a regular practice rather than something that only happens when there is a problem, they are far more likely to be receptive. When coaching or feedback is unexpected, or it is something team members aren't accustomed to, there can be resistance. If coaching hasn't been the norm, leaders who introduce coaching must effectively prepare members for the coaching process by explaining the purpose and what they can expect.

Words have different connotations for different people. If you suspect that *coaching* is a word that might have negative connotations for some members of your team, you might instead call it "mentoring" or whatever you feel would be effective language.

There are a number of ways that coaching can be useful. For example, it might support a developmental need that you have recognized because of a specific incident, or from the results of a team assessment that members completed as part of the team development process. It can also be part of an ongoing performance-management process for your team members. When coaching is tied to a specific situation the process is most effective if it is introduced as soon as possible after the event. For example, in a team meeting you might notice that one team member consistently puts down the ideas of others without taking the time to listen fully to their points of view. Taking time right after the meeting to capitalize on this coaching opportunity will be more effective than waiting a month to do so.

For these coaching opportunities to be identified, the leader must be circulating, observing, and participating. It is easy to allow oneself to be glued to one's desk. With an increased amount of administrative work, for instance, a unit manager can become heads-down focused, with their desk becoming a barrier between themselves and the world of their team and patients. Once trapped there, it can take great effort to change personal routine, behaviour, and organization to get out and about.

Clinical near-miss events and errors present easy-to-identify coaching needs. However, leaders, particularly those who are not naturally process oriented, may not as readily notice the important coaching opportunities that unproductive behaviours (for example, an inappropriate interaction with a team member or response to a patient) present. Leaders also may more readily ignore personal behaviours because they are seen as more sensitive issues and more difficult to address. Ignoring them is dangerous. Behavioural issues can directly affect the quality of patient care in the same way that clinical issues can. Indirectly, they affect patient care by contributing to a negative team climate in which neither the team member nor the patient thrives.

THE COACHING PROCESS

The attitude that leaders take with them into the coaching process sets the tone and, to a great extent, determines the results. Coaching is not about the leader as an authority figure telling a team member what he or she needs to do differently. At its best, the coaching process is a shared responsibility and experience: the coach and team member work together to ensure the member learns and brings forward his or her very best.

Coaches look for opportunities to ask questions rather than direct or give orders. As much as possible, they help the person they're coaching to identify and/or change unproductive practices and behaviours, or to develop skills needed to excel. However, the effective coaching style is a balanced one in which the leader knows when it is best to pose questions and when it is best to give directions. The leader as coach, for instance, uses a "telling" or "explaining" mode when he or she establishes expectations or explains a clinical procedure.

Coaching includes the following:

- Establishing developmental goals
- Clarifying performance expectations
- Providing feedback
- Probing for a greater understanding of the member being coached or of his or her level of knowledge and ability
- Asking questions that assist the member being coached in his or her own self discovery
- Providing advice
- Celebrating growth and success stories

The atmosphere is informal, but the coaching conversation, however short, has structure whether it is taking place on the floor, at the bedside, or in an office. An effective coaching conversation requires that

- The objectives for the conversation are clear
- A specific issue, practice, skill, or behaviour is discussed
- Agreements on changes that need to be made or worked toward are set
- Key points are recapped by either the coach or person they're coaching

The coaching process includes three phases:

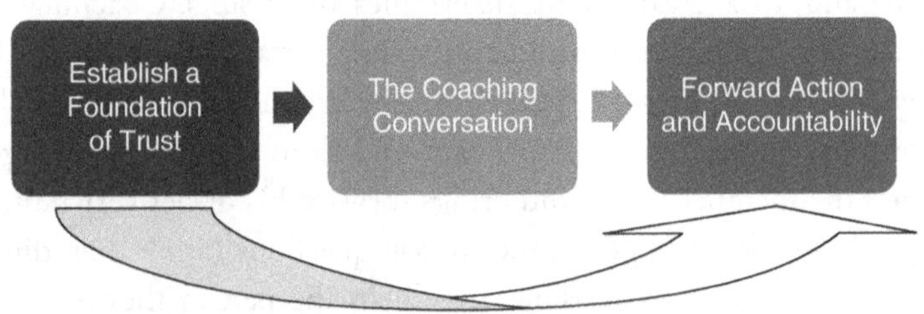

Figure 12.1: The Coaching Process

ESTABLISH A FOUNDATION OF TRUST

It is mutual trust and respect that create an enduring coaching relationship. This is essential whether you are embarking upon a formal coaching relationship or coaching spontaneously and in the moment. An effective leader strives to create a positive environment for the team member so that he or she will be open and receptive to being coached. The team member's perception of the leader's desire to help will determine whether or not the coaching is successful.

As was discussed in Chapter 2: Climate: A Cornerstone of the Staff and Patient Experience, building trust is dependent upon a number of components, including walking the talk, behaving consistently, and showing concern for the well-being of others. An essential aspect of each of these trust-building components is the leader's ability to listen attentively. When a leader effectively practices the art of listening, and gives his or her full attention to another, the leader will demonstrate a desire to understand and support the individual he or she is interacting with and therefore will create greater trust.

The Art of Listening: The Three S's

Listening is an active process that requires participation on the part of the listener. Attentive listening means listening without distraction and ensuring the other person knows you are interested and engaged in what they have to say.

Attentive listening requires that the listener demonstrate each of the following *three s's* during conversations:

Show empathy and acknowledge feelings.
Seek clarification (while withholding judgment).
Summarize.

Show Empathy and Acknowledge Feelings

Showing empathy requires that you understand the perspective of the speaker by mentally stepping into his or her shoes. It may sound like the speaker wants you to agree with him, but in reality he mainly wants you to understand his feelings and point of view.

Showing empathy and acknowledging feelings requires that you not only take in the words of the speaker, but also look at the whole message being sent, including body language, tone of voice, and level of emotion. Together these communicate the emotion the speaker is feeling. You can then let the speaker know that you realize he or she is feeling a particular emotion by acknowledging it in one sentence.

For example:

"I understand you feel you are not being *heard.*"
"I can see how important *respect* is to you."
"I can see that this situation is causing you a lot of *stress.*"
"I can understand why you felt *condescended* to and *put down.*"

It is helpful to incorporate verbal and non-verbal cues to acknowledge the speaker. These could include nodding your head, leaning in, using appropriate facial expressions to convey empathy, and commenting "yes," "mmhmm," and so on to show you are actively listening.

Seek Clarification (While Withholding Judgment)

To convey that you are making an effort to understand the speaker, use questions and probe for more information. To formulate a relevant question when asking for more clarification, you will have to listen carefully to what is being said. Frame your question in a way that allows you to understand in more detail what is being said. Asking for a specific example can be useful. This also helps the speaker to evaluate his or her own opinions and perspectives.

"Can you give me an example . . ."
"Tell me a little more about . . ."

Summarize

Reiterate the speaker's message back to him or her to confirm that you understand what's been said. Summarizing involves using your own words to paraphrase what the speaker has said without judging its validity or merit, and getting confirmation that you understood the message correctly.

For example:

"What I'm hearing from you is that you'd like to . . ."
"If I understand you correctly, you feel that . . ."
"You'd like to find a way to resolve the conflict you are having with Susan in a manner that won't harm your working relationship, is that right?"

The Coaching Conversation

Coaching happens through conversations. Whether the conversations are formal or informal, the purpose is to

- Support the team member's development as it relates to specific growth opportunities in behavior, skill, and attitude through feedback, challenging of the member's thinking or mind set, and knowledge sharing
- Develop a clear picture of what will be different when the member is performing at their best
- Develop a plan for closing the gap

Table 12.1 provides a five-step process for structuring the coaching conversation and provides examples of the types of questions that can be asked during each step of the process. Leaders who use this model during either formal or informal conversations will find that while it may take more time at the outset, practicing the technique will save time in the long run. Importantly, it prevents conversations that produce nonproductive outcomes; the conversation will end with clear solutions and next steps. Table 12.1 has been adapted from the GROW model—originally conceived by Graham Alexander and John Whitmore—which is used extensively throughout the field of coaching.

Table 12.1: I-Grow: A Model for Structuring the Coaching

Issue	*What's up?*	Identify the current issue (e.g., performance related, behavioural, task, skill, interpersonal.)
Goal	*What do you want?*	Define what the team member wants or needs to achieve.

(continued)

Reality	*What's happening now?*	Explore the current situation. What is the gap between where they are now and where they want to be? Once the team member has provided his/her assessment of the situation, you can provide feedback.
Options	*What could you do?*	Help the team member to identify ideas, solutions, and options for achieving the goal/addressing the issue. Then you can offer additional options/advice.
Way Forward	*What will you do?*	The team member commits to specific actions.

Identify the Issue: "What's up?"

The issue is often fairly evident, in particular when the leader has identified an on-the-job coachable moment related to a skill, task, or behaviour. The leader's opener can determine the quality of the coaching moment. Examples of coaching openers can be found in Table 12.2.

On other occasions, the issue may not be immediately evident. For example, you might notice that a new nursing graduate is visibly upset after speaking with a physician. Since you did not witness the interaction between the nurse and the physician, you do not know what the issue is. In this instance, you might begin the coaching conversation with the following opener: "I can see that you are a little frazzled after speaking with Dr. Smith. I know how tough it can be to communicate with some of the staff—what happened?"

Table 12.2: Examples of Coaching Openers

"I know how challenging it can be to communicate assertively and clearly with some team members. Let's talk about what you can do to improve your communication."
"Let's talk about how you can more accurately assess this type of case."
"Would you like me to help you to . . .?"
"I've experienced this situation many times; would you like to talk about how you can . . .?"

Establish a Goal: "What Do You Want?"

Once the issue has been identified, turn it into a positive goal statement that clearly communicates what the individual would like to achieve. It is at this stage that the right questions can change the individual's issue into a goal. Once the individual embraces the importance of achieving the goal, his or her engagement, commitment, and motivation are increased. Their focus is shifted from a potentially de-motivating and stressful issue to an opportunity to excel and grow. Next, the leader can help the individual develop a clear and concise goal that can be measured so that both the individual and leader will know when the goal has been achieved. The purpose of establishing a goal is to help the individual to

- Articulate exactly what they want to achieve.
- Identify why the goal is important.
- Identify how the goal will be measured.
- Set a time frame for achieving the goal.

Table 12.3 provides a list of questions a leader can use when helping a team member set goals.

Table 12.3: Goal-Setting Questions

"What do you want to achieve?"
"What would the ideal outcome be?"
"What areas do you want to strengthen, grow, develop?"
"What will be different once you achieve the goal?"
"How will achieving the goal help you, your team, your patients?"
"How will you know when you have achieved your goal?"
"What are you doing that shows you have achieved your goal?"
"How will you feel when you've achieved your goal?"

Explore Reality: "What's Happening Now?"

This phase focuses on gaining a better understanding of the specific situation and the current reality of the individual. It is during this phase that the leader can begin to provide constructive feedback based on his or her observations and experience. However, an effective coach will refrain from providing feedback until the individual has had the opportunity to fully explore the situation and evaluate himself or herself with the help of the coach's questions.

1. Gain Insight: Dig Deeper into the Need/Issue/Goal

The first step of exploring reality is to understand the current situation in relation to the issue or goal. The questions in Table 12.4 not only help the leader gain greater clarity, they also provide the opportunity for the individual to reflect more deeply on the issue and/or goal. This gives him or her a better grasp of how to effectively achieve the goal, or it could bring an entirely new perspective to the issue.

Table 12.4: Questions for Exploring Reality

"Would you describe the situation for me?"
"What is happening now that tells you that you have an issue or problem?"
"What is likely to occur if the issue isn't resolved/if you don't change/improve/ achieve your goal?"
"What have you done so far to improve things?"
"Where are you now in relation to your goal?"
"On a scale of one to ten—one being very far from achieving your goal and ten being very close—how close are you to achieving your goal?"
"What has contributed to your success so far?"
"What skills/knowledge/attributes do you have that will help you achieve this goal?"

2. Share Observations and Provide Constructive Feedback

Once the team member has had the opportunity to reflect on the current situation, the leader provides feedback based on his or her observations and experience. This is particularly effective if the leader has observed the team member "in action," demonstrating the behaviours and skills that the member would like to improve.

Steps to Providing Constructive Feedback

Describe the facts about the problem/issue as you know it.

1. Base your description on what you have observed, not on your interpretation and opinion.

When the facts you want to describe relate to the team member's behaviours, ensure that you are describing visible behaviours; otherwise, it is just your perception, and your comments will sound judgmental and the other person can easily argue them.

X "You don't listen to our patients."

This statement describes a behaviour that is not visible (listening). It is a judgmental statement that is based on one person's interpretation of an event or events. This statement could lead to a defensive response.

✔ "I notice that when a patient is speaking with you, you don't make eye contact with them. Instead, you are reading their chart, or are occupied doing something else."

This statement describes the facts—specific, observed behaviours, and not an interpretation of the events as shown above.

2. Elaborate on/explain why the behaviour is a problem.

   The individual may have already identified how the behaviour is impacting the team, their performance, the patient, and so on. If so, recap what the individual has said. If not, explain why the behaviour is a problem.

   "When you don't stop what you are doing to make eye contact with patients, it can be perceived as not listening and as not caring about their needs. One of our unit's objectives is to improve our patients' experience; maintaining eye contact with them when they're speaking with you helps ensure that they feel you're listening to them and that their needs are your priority."

3. Invite dialogue/the other person's point of view.

   Use phrases such as: "What do you think?" and "Tell me, what are your thoughts?"

Identify Options: "What Could You Do?"

In this stage, the goal is not to immediately find a solution, but to generate possible alternative courses of action. Before offering input, the most effective coach allows the individual the opportunity to identify his or her own options or solutions. For leaders who are more task oriented, this may take practice because their own tendency is likely to prescribe a solution rather than encourage the person they are coaching to identify options on his or her own.

Table 12.5 provides a list of questions the leader can use when identifying options.

Table 12.5: Questions for the Options Phase

"What could you do to move yourself just one step forward?"
"What are your options?"
"Give me five options."
"What could you do differently?"
"What have you tried so far?"
"How have you tackled a similar situation before?"
"What worked, what didn't, what did you learn?"
"What do you believe you need to do differently?"
"What could you do if fear were not a factor?"
"What could you do if, no matter what happened, everyone said, 'Well done for trying'?"
"What haven't you tried that might let you move yourself one step closer?"
"What are the pros and cons of each option?"
"What do you have control over?"
"What resources do you have/need?"

The Way Forward: "What Will You Do?"

In this last step the leader assists the team member in choosing an option (or options) with which to move forward, and helps them set a concrete plan of action. It is essential that the conversation end with the individual identifying at least one commitment to action for achieving their goal and/or addressing the issue at hand.

Table 12.6 provides a list of questions the leader can use to help guide the team member.

Table 12.6: Taking Action to Move Forward

"Which option would best take you to your goal?"
"Tell me specifically what actions you will take and when you will take them."
"What exactly will you do to reach your goal, and when?"
"Which of these options will you move forward with?"
"What concrete step can you take now?"
"What steps come after?"
"When will you do this?"
"How will this plan get you to your goal?"
"How can I help you?"
"How can I help you stay accountable to your commitment?"

FORWARD ACTION AND ACCOUNTABILITY

The leader's role continues after the coaching conversation ends, and includes providing team members with encouragement, support, and establishing accountability for performance improvement. Incorporating the following coaching "best practices" will assist you in modeling positive behaviours while helping to ensure your team members remain engaged and motivated.

- ✔ **Check-in regularly:** Develop the habit of having open conversations with your team members. Make a conscious effort to find time everyday to connect. This not only builds trust and promotes open communication, but also provides the opportunity to informally check in on how your team members are progressing in achieving the goals they identified.
- ✔ **Keep track of goals and timelines:** When a team member sets a specific goal with a specific timeline, check back in to ensure the member is on track. This provides another opportunity to have a coaching conversation in case the individual is encountering any barriers to achieving their goal. This also lets the individual know that the goals he or she has set will not be forgotten, and that the team member is held accountable for achieving them.

✔ **Provide feedback:** Develop the habit of providing both positive and constructive feedback. Look for opportunities to reinforce positive behaviour, especially when an individual is making progress toward achieving a goal. Look for opportunities to provide constructive feedback that will help the individual continue to progress toward his or her goals. This will let the individual know you are committed to his or her development and professional growth.

POINTS TO REMEMBER FOR MAKING IT HAPPEN

A multi-pronged approach to the team development process builds the most effective teams. A successful team development process should include the following:

- Providing strong leadership
- Conducting team assessments
- Exhibiting the strong facilitation skills, required to lead effective team meetings and development sessions
- Using coaching skills to assist individual team members in strengthening their contribution to the team

Adopting and committing to such a process will prod, challenge, and support the team in what will be an exciting and transforming growth experience.

Part III

The Tools to Make It Happen

13

Team Development Exercises

In Parts I and II, we covered a lot of ground in terms of the ingredients required for agile, collaborative, and patient-focused teams and leadership attitude, skills, and practices that ensure these essentials are alive and well. In Part III we provide team development exercises, which we refer to as *workouts*, that are designed to strengthen each of the seven essential team elements that we have described. These workouts will get teams into shape and sustain the level of fitness required to be a high-performing team. The exercises provide the framework for team dialogue and learning, and support the kind of breakthroughs in thinking and relationships that lead to stronger, patient-focused teams.

Each workout can stand alone and be incorporated into a team meeting, a "lunch and learn," or a team huddle. Or, several activities can be woven together to create a team development workshop. The workouts are designed to provide the support you need to create and facilitate team development, which will bring about exceptional change whether you are an experienced professional or a novice facilitator. We have included a variety of activities. Each will trigger important discussion and result in teams developing commitments to action for change and growth.

HOW THIS PART IS STRUCTURED

We'll begin this part of the book with two exercises that focus on overall team development and the maintenance of commitments to action and agreements that are made to improve team performance.

In the second part of this section, we'll provide team development exercises designed to strengthen each of the seven elements of high-performance teams, along with short brainteaser activities that can be used at the beginning of team meetings to bring the team together and spark creative thinking.

The exercises, associated handouts, and PowerPoint slides can be found at www.healthcareteamperformance.com along with additional resources to help ensure that your team development process runs as smoothly as possible.

WORKOUTS

WORKOUT 1: CLARIFYING EXPECTATIONS

Time Required: *30 minutes to 1 hour depending on size of team and length of discussion.*

Objective

To develop a better understanding of one another's needs and to commit to making an effort to meet these needs.

Background

If morale is low or there is conflict within the team, it is often because the team has not taken time to explore the needs of its individual members. Team members may be hurt or frustrated because their expectations are not being met. Frequently, however, these expectations have not been articulated, and others are either unaware of them or do not understand the importance the team member has attached to them. Expectations are often based on personal needs.

This workout can start team development, energize members when they are showing signs of discontent or lethargy, or strengthen the team's climate element. If used as a team development starting point in lieu of a team assessment, keep in mind that the outcomes of the workout will not be as detailed with respect to its growth opportunities. Also, because the exercise necessitates that team members ask fellow members to discuss their needs of one another, members must be comfortable speaking openly, and the facilitator requires the skills to enable them to create a comfortable environment.

Clarifying expectations is a powerful activity that can quickly enhance team climate and cohesiveness.

Materials Required:

- Flip chart

Steps

1. Select one of the following incomplete statements to act as a thought trigger for participants.

"In order to give my best to the team, I need my teammates to..."
or
"I believe we would be a more effective team if team members..."

2. Post the statement on a flip chart and ask participants to complete the statement independently. Inform the team members they can complete the statement as many times as they need to in order to clarify all of their needs. Note: Expectations identified are usually basic needs that can be quite easily met by other team members.
3. Ask team members to share their statements.

COMMON RESPONSES

I need my team members to...

- Keep me better informed.
- Be more readily available to help me out when I am swamped and they are not busy.
- Be open to me asking them questions.
- Ask me for my opinion.

4. Discuss each of the statements. You might choose to use the following questions to structure the discussion.

ASK Is this a realistic expectation?

If the answer is yes:

ASK Is there anything preventing anyone from living up to [name of team member]'s expectation?

If the answer is no:

ASK **Is everyone then prepared to make a commitment to meet this need?**

Note: If the team or any member feels that they cannot live up to a team member's need, this may lead to awareness that a team member holds an unrealistic expectation. It may also present an opportunity for the team to look for a creative solution: what else might be done to solve this team member's concern?

Encourage follow-through by asking:

ASK How can you ensure that team members live up to these commitments?

COMMON RESPONSE

- We must each make a personal commitment to do so.
- The person who has expressed a particular need must remind us if we are slipping.
- Everyone must be receptive to reminders if we are not living up to a commitment.

5. Turn the agreed upon responses into a set of team agreements. For example, a set of team agreements based on the possible responses described above might be as follows:

   We agree to
   - Keep one another better informed
   - Be ready to help out when people are swamped
   - Be open to people asking us questions
   - Ask team members for their input

   We will ensure we live up to these agreements by
   - Taking personal responsibility for doing so
   - Letting others know when they are failing to meet an expectation that we have identified
   - Being receptive when a team member reminds us that we have slipped in meeting an expectation that they have identified

WORKOUT 2: MAINTAINING TEAM FITNESS

Time Required: *15 minutes*

Objective

To ensure follow-through on commitments to action made by the team.

Background

This workout is to be used as a follow-up to the team workouts listed in this chapter as a means to maintain momentum and to keep team development top of mind. Book 15 minutes at the beginning of at least one team meeting a month to check on team development progress and to reinforce commitments to action made during previous team development exercises. Depending on how far along you are in the development process, and the number of commitments to action the team has made, you may review them all or select a few (perhaps four or five) that the team has identified as particularly important.

Keep in mind that, for high-performance teams, team development is an ongoing process. The strongest teams regularly check how they are doing. It is recommended that you make this practice an ongoing habit.

Materials Required

- A list of team commitments to action made during the previous team development exercise(s)

Steps

1. Review commitments to action. For each commitment to action, ask the following questions to trigger discussion:

ASK	How well are we living up to this commitment?

ASK	Can you give an example of how we are living up to this commitment?

Or, if the group doesn't feel they are living up to the commitment:

ASK Can you give an example of how we have slipped with this commitment?

ASK Is there a reason we're having trouble living up to this commitment?

ASK Can we renew our commitment to this one?

2. Recap. When reviewing outcomes of the discussion, you might say:

SAY We have agreed that we are doing really well with _______, but we need to make a greater effort to _______.

WORKOUT 3: IT'S ALL ABOUT RESPECT

Element strengthened: Healthy Climate

Time Required: *45 minutes to 1 hour.*

Objective

To strengthen the team climate by increasing members' respect for one another.

Materials Required

- Sheets of red and green paper (one sheet of each colour per team member)
- Tape

Steps

1. Share the definition of *respect* as shown below (it is recommended that you write it on a flip chart).

   Respect: To show, through your behaviour, that you value an individual.

2. Ask members to think about behaviours that demonstrate respect, and behaviours that demonstrate lack of respect.
3. Ask participants to write on their red sheet of paper one behaviour that they believe is disrespectful and that they would like to see stopped.
4. Ask participants to write on their green sheet of paper one behaviour that they believe demonstrates respect and that they would like to see more often.
5. Put the headings "STOP" and "START" on a board or wall. Ask members to post their red sheets under the heading "STOP," and green under the heading "START."
6. Facilitate a discussion of each behaviour identified.

When discussing the "red behaviours," you might ask:

ASK Why do people at times behave in these ways?

When discussing the "green behaviours," you might ask:

ASK Why don't people behave this way more often?

7. Facilitate agreement on two or three behaviours that team members will stop, and two or three behaviours that team members will put into practice.
8. Ask the group to identify how they will keep each other accountable for living up to these behaviours. What should the next steps be?
9. Recap behaviours and next steps, and have the group reconfirm its commitment.

WORKOUT 4: JUMPING TO CONCLUSIONS

Element strengthened: *Healthy Climate*

Time Required: *40 minutes*

Objective

To strengthen the climate element by learning the steps to managing personal assumptions, and by allowing participants the opportunity to identify assumptions—about themselves or other team members—that are impeding their ability to develop positive relationships.

Background

Assumptions are very often at the heart of conflict and poor interpersonal relationships. The challenge in managing assumptions is that we don't know when we're making them. They come from our own paradigms (our firm ideas about what is right and what is wrong). Paradigms come from our past experience, our culture, and our upbringing. If someone is behaving in a way that does not fit our personal paradigms, we may make assumptions about that person, discount them, or choose not to interact with them.

For example, if a team member is boastful, but we have been brought up to believe that one should be modest, the member's behaviour may turn us off, and we may miss what the member has to contribute. Another assumption we may hold is that silence means disagreement. In this case, if we are taking part in the discussion of an important change, and one team member is not contributing, we may interpret this as a lack of support for the change.

We also hold assumptions about ourselves, which influence our interpretation of people's behaviour toward us. For example, if we feel inadequate in any way, we may interpret someone else's behaviour toward us as being critical, when that was not the intent. Our personal fears may also cause us to misinterpret others' actions.

Assumptions cause us to jump to conclusions. When there is conflict or poor interpersonal relationships, it is important that members are able to monitor themselves and check whether their feelings and reactions are based on fact or assumption.

Materials Required

None

Steps

1. Share the following story.

   Donna and Jim were concerned about staff scheduling over the upcoming holidays. They felt that instead of their manager developing the schedule on his own, the team should work together to create a schedule that would work for everyone. After discussing it over coffee, they decided to raise the issue in the next meeting with their manager. In the corridor of their workplace, they bumped into their team member Janet, and told her their plan. They asked if she agreed, and if she would support them in the meeting. She said that it was definitely an important issue and promised to support them.

   During the meeting, Jim raised the issue. However, the manager quickly dismissed it, even though Donna said that she supported Jim's idea. Janet said nothing and left quickly after the meeting. Donna and Jim were not happy. Over the next few days, the more they talked about it, the angrier they became.

2. Generate a discussion:

   ASK If you were Donna or Jim, what would you conclude?

   COMMON RESPONSES

   - We can't count on Janet.
   - Janet was afraid to speak up.
   - Janet is not someone I would count on again.

3. Explain what actually happened.

   Just prior to the meeting, Janet received word that her father was seriously ill. Throughout the meeting, she was distracted by the news, and she rushed off to see her father as soon as the meeting was finished.

ASK Does this additional information change your conclusions?

SAY Donna and Jim—and many of us—were making assumptions. We came to a conclusion without the facts.

4. Write the following definition of *assumptions* on a flip chart:

   Coming to a conclusion not based on fact.

5. Share information from the Background section of this workout, and then return to the story of Janet.

ASK What paradigms or beliefs could have influenced Donna and Jim, causing them to immediately react without checking for facts or giving Janet the benefit of the doubt?

COMMON RESPONSES

- A strong belief that a person should always follows through on their commitments.
- A belief that you should always be able to count on your friends.
- A belief that people are liable to wimp out if they think that speaking up about an issue will negatively affect how management sees them.

6. Explain that there are negative beliefs as well as positive ones that generally stand us in good stead. However, if we use our beliefs to jump to conclusions without first checking facts, then we are making assumptions.

7. Ask members to identify assumptions they see their team making. For example, we may think that a doctor who is being abrupt is putting us down. Or, if a team member doesn't respond the way that we do to a sensitive issue, we may assume he or she doesn't care.
   If there are more than seven members of your team, break into small discussion groups. If your team has seven or fewer members, have people work in pairs or triads.
8. Invite members to share examples of assumptions that the team has made, and ask, "In what ways are these assumptions limiting you or creating problems?"
9. Explain that it takes vigilance to manage our assumptions, because often we don't realize we are making them. It requires self-discipline to frequently check for assumptions. It can be beneficial, if members are receptive, to kindly point out to one another when assumptions are being made.
10. Ask the members how they feel they can best manage their assumptions, and facilitate agreement on assumption-management actions.

WORKOUT 5: VALUES CHECK

Element strengthened: *Cohesiveness*

Time Required: *45 minutes to 1.5 hours*
Note: This can be presented in one longer activity or two shorter ones.

Objective

To strengthen team cohesiveness by assessing the degree to which team members demonstrate key team values, and by increasing team members' commitment to consistently demonstrating those values.

Background

High-performance teams are clear about *who* they are as well as *what* they do. Many different teams perform many of the same tasks. What makes a team unique is *how* it approaches its tasks. Team values determine the *how*. To be useful, values must be appropriate to the team's mission and goals, and therefore must be examined within that context.

Materials Required

- Handouts (2), which are included here and can also be found at www.healthcareteamperformance.com

Steps

1. Post the team's values in a visible place. If the team has not yet developed a set of team values, complete the following steps:
   a. Choose one of the following:
      - Post the team's mission statement if one has already been developed.
      - Post the team's goals.
      - Lead the team in the development of a "success statement" that describes what success looks like to the team (e.g., "Success is improving patient satisfaction by 20 per cent in two years").

   b. Develop a list of four or five values that team members believe they must consistently demonstrate if they are to meet their mission or goals, or fulfill their success statement. Examples of values frequently identified as important include responsiveness, quality, commitment, and teamwork.

Note: If time is an issue, the above step can be conducted as a separate workout, to be followed by steps 2 to 8 (below) at a later time.

2. Provide each team member with a copy of the worksheets "Demonstrating Team Values" and "Team Commitments to Action" (Handouts A and B).
3. Ask members to assess the demonstration of their team values by completing the "Demonstrating Team Values" worksheet. Allow approximately 10 minutes.
4. Ask team members to share their assessment of each value.
5. Agree on which values are consistently demonstrated and which need more attention.
6. For each value that requires more attention, develop a team list of actions that need to be taken or behaviours that need to be demonstrated.
7. Ask team members to commit to taking the actions they have agreed upon in order to strengthen the values.
8. Ask members to recap these commitments on the "Team Commitments to Action" worksheet provided, and to refer back to it regularly.

DEMONSTRATING TEAM VALUES

Handout A

Participant's Worksheet

Values	**Rate how well you believe the value is currently demonstrated (scale of 1 to 10: 1 is low and 10 is high).**	**List what you believe the team should do *more* of to strengthen the value.**	**List what you believe the team should do *less* of to strengthen the value.**

Handout
Page 2 of 2

TEAM COMMITMENTS TO ACTION

Handout B

Value: ________________

In order to strengthen this value, we will:

Value: ________________

In order to strengthen this value, we will:

Value: ________________

In order to strengthen this value, we will:

Value: ________________

In order to strengthen this value, we will:

Value: ________________

In order to strengthen this value, we will:

WORKOUT 6: WE'RE ALL IN THIS TOGETHER

Element Strengthened: *Cohesiveness*

Time Required: *45 minutes to 1 hour*

Objective

To strengthen the Cohesiveness element by identifying the behaviours related to hierarchy that impact the team members' ability to work effectively together.

Materials Required

- Handout: "We're All in This Together" which is included here and can also be found at www.healthcareteamperformance.com
- Coloured sticky dots
- Flip charts

Steps

1. For large teams, break the team into smaller groups of four to six.
2. Distribute the "We're All in This Together" handout and review the instructions. Ask that the groups capture their ideas on a flip chart.
3. Invite groups to share their ideas.
4. Assist the group in reaching a consensus on the top three to five recommendations they will implement and/or commit to (from question 3 on the handout).

   For teams that develop a long list of recommendations, you can prioritize the list by asking participants to place dots next to the items that, in their experience, are most important.

   Give each participant the number of dots that equals 20 per cent of the total number of items on the list. For example, if there are 10 items on the list, each participant is given two dots; if there are 20 items, each participant is given four dots, etc.

   The participants can use their dots however they choose. For example, if they have two dots, they can place both dots against the item they feel most strongly about, or they can place one dot next to each of their top two choices. The three to five recommendations that receive the most number of votes (dots) are the items the team will move forward with.

5. Recap the top three to five recommendations and confirm commitment.
6. Identify what the team will do to ensure that the recommendations are implemented, and establish a means for follow-up.

Handout
Page 1 of 1

WE'RE ALL IN THIS TOGETHER

1. Identify behaviours and/or examples that indicate that hierarchy is impacting your team's cohesiveness.

____

____

____

____

____

2. Identify the ways in which these behaviours impact your team's cohesiveness and your ability to perform at your best.

____

____

____

____

____

3. Complete the following sentence: "In order to help ensure that hierarchy in our team does not impact our cohesiveness, we need to…"

____

____

____

____

____

Be prepared to share with the larger group.

WORKOUT 7: THE PRINCIPLES OF EFFECTIVE COMMUNICATION

Element strengthened: *Open Communication*

Time Required: 20 minutes to 1.5 hours

Note: The four principles of effective communication can be presented as a 1 to 1.5-hour workshop, as presented below, or you may present the principles separately in mini meetings of 20 to 30 minutes.

Objective

To strengthen the open communication element by:

- Discovering communication issues within the team
- Understanding the principles of effective communication
- Identifying team goals for improved communication

Background

Communication skills affect every aspect of team effectiveness, interpersonal relationships, quality of patient care, and performance at work. Communicating effectively is a skill that requires knowledge, time, and practice to develop to its full potential. Many teams and individuals are unable to work at high levels of performance because the fundamental communication knowledge and know-how are missing.

The communication principles outlined in this exercise are relatively easy to grasp and understand. However, if they are not applied consistently, they will be of little to no benefit to the team. In this exercise, the team members identify the specific barriers currently present in their team that are preventing them from communicating effectively. They use the knowledge gained through the session to determine what they will do to remove, or, at the very least, weaken the barriers.

Materials Required

- Sheets of paper (at least 8 1/2" × 11" (215 mm × 279 mm)) and felt-tip marker or crayon for each member.
- PowerPoint slides: PrinciplesofEffectiveCommunicationSlides.ppt found at www.healthcareteamperformance.com
- Flip chart

Steps

1. Introduce the exercise by linking it to the team's needs.
2. Distribute sheets of paper (at least 8 1/2" × 11" (215 mm × 279 mm) in size) and felt-tip markers or crayons.
3. Ensure participants are seated far enough apart to allow them to work privately.
4. Ask participants to individually identify the biggest barrier to open communication in the team, and to write it as briefly as possible in large letters on their sheet of paper. Then have them fold the paper.

COMMON RESPONSES

- People not listening
- Lack of respect for each other's opinions
- Fear of repercussions
- Wanting to avoid conflict

5. Post the collected responses on a board or wall. With help from the group, organize similar points under common headings.
6. Review the responses and ask the team for comments and observations regarding what the team has identified as key barriers to open communication.
7. Ask team members to comment on how poor communication impacts their team's effectiveness.
8. Share the following:

SAY We will spend a good portion of today's session identifying what you as a team can do to remove each of these barriers so that you can communicate more effectively with one another. Before we do that, however, let's spend some time reviewing the principles of effective communication.

ASK There are four principles of effective communication. What do you think they are?

Capture responses on the flip chart.

9. Show slide 2 in PrinciplesofEffectiveCommunicationSlides.ppt, and share the four principles with the team.
10. Introduce Principle 1: Listen, Really Listen (slide 3). Prior to displaying the bullet points on the slide, generate a discussion:

SAY	"Listen, Really Listen" is the first principle. Let's spend some time reviewing the behaviours and practices of an active listener.

ASK	How do you know when someone is listening effectively?

Capture responses on the flip chart.

11. Review each point on slide 3, linking the points to the participants' ideas, which you captured on the flip chart. Key information to share as a wrap-up of this principle:

SAY	Listening is not simply waiting for your turn to talk. Listening is a choice made with the intent of truly understanding what the other person is saying. First, decide that you will listen, and then listen with a clean slate.

12. Introduce Principle 2: Respond Instead of React (slide 4). Prior to displaying the bullet points on the slide, generate a discussion:

SAY	"Respond Instead of React" is the second principle. What do you think this means?

Capture responses on the flip chart.

13. Review each point on slide 4, linking the points to the participants' ideas, which you captured on the flip chart.
14. Introduce Principle 3: Ask Questions to Clarify (slide 5). Prior displaying the bullet points on the slide, generate a discussion:

ASK	What is the purpose of asking questions?

COMMON RESPONSES

- To let the individual know you are listening and are interested.
- To clarify understanding and to challenge assumptions that the listener might have.
- To build a rapport.

15. Recap this principle by reviewing each point on slide 5, linking the points to the participants' ideas, which you captured on the flip chart.
16. Introduce Principle 4: Recap Understanding (slide 6). Prior to displaying the bullet points on the slide, generate a discussion:

ASK Why is it important to recap understanding?

Capture responses on the flip chart.

17. Review each point on slide 6, linking the points to the participants' ideas, which you captured on the flip chart.
18. Recap the four principles and ask if the participants have any questions.
19. Return to the barriers to open communication that the group identified at the beginning of the session, and identify the three barriers that were most common among the team members.
20. Discuss each barrier, looking for ways to remove it:

SAY Some of you are concerned about _____. Given what we have learned today, and what you know about your team, what can you do to remove this barrier and improve your communication?

Capture responses on the flip chart.

21. Reach a consensus on the top three or four things the team can do to improve its communication effectiveness.

ASK If everyone lives up to these commitments, is it agreed that this barrier will be removed or at least weakened?

22. End this exercise by recapping commitments to action and identifying how team members will keep each other accountable to their commitments.

WORKOUT 8: MAKE YOUR VOICE COUNT

***Element strengthened:** Open Communication*

***Time Required:** 45 minutes to 1 hour*

Objective

To strengthen the open communication element by helping team members recognize that the way we approach others affects whether or not our point of view will be heard.

Background

It is often said that the definition of insanity is doing the same thing over and over again and expecting a different result. If we repeatedly get a response from others that is not what we had hoped for, we need to assess how we are presenting ourselves and our ideas. Often we put the blame on the other. Instead, self reflection is called for. Do we need to approach people differently or express ourselves differently? In addition to our words, does our body language affect how what we put forward is received?

Our ideas and points of view can't count and we can't make our maximum contribution if we are not heard. If we don't feel we are being heard the first step in getting people's positive attention is to change our approach.

Materials Required

- A flip chart for each discussion group
- Handout: "It's All in the Approach" which is included here and can also be found at www.healthcareteamperformance.com

Steps

1. Generate discussion with the following:

> **SAY** Open communication is an element that you/we have identified as an opportunity for improvement. For there to be open communication, it is essential that everyone's voice be heard.
>
> Whether our voice is heard depends on whether we speak up and on how we do that. Let's consider both of these.
>
> If we speak up we, of course, can't be heard. Most of us have experiences in which we would like to speak up but don't. In your experience, what causes people not to speak up if they have an idea or concern?

Allow a minute of reflection time and then capture responses on a flip chart or white board. Allow two to three minutes of discussion.

Note: This type of discussion can lend itself to venting. While venting can be positive, and is at times necessary in order to move toward solutions, be sure that the venting does not last too long and that the objective of the discussion is not lost.

> **COMMON RESPONSES**
>
> - We think the other person won't be responsive. They may see it as criticism.
> - We think the other person is busy or stressed.
> - We have been shot down before—sometimes in front of the patient.

Capture Responses

Note: Some responses may not be based on fact. They may be assumptions or generalizations such as: "Doctors don't respect us" or "Doctors don't care what we think." When you receive responses that are assumptions or generalizations, it presents an opportunity to challenge these assumptions. Ask (respectfully and in an open manner), "How do you know that to be true?" Capture responses on the flip chart.

2. Distribute the "It's All About the Approach" handout and review the instructions. Ask members to work in groups of 4 or 5 to complete the activity.

> **SAY** Now let's think about our approach and how important it is to the way in which our input is received.

3. Ask groups to share the ideas generated from the activity and capture them so that they are visible to the group.
4. Identify the top three ideas that the group agrees to commit to. Ask for commitment from the group to live up to these ideas going forward.

   Note: If the group creates a long agreed upon list, ask them to select the top three or four to begin with. Ensure, however, that you revisit the commitments in the near future to both check how well members are living up to them and also to add additional commitments from their original list.

Handout
Page 1 of 1

ITS ALL IN THE APPROACH

As a group, respond to the questions below and capture your responses on a flip chart. Be prepared to share your responses with the larger group.

1. Please take a few minutes of quiet time. If some members complete the following individual assignment before others please respect them by remaining quiet.

   Individual assignment: Individually consider how one's approach affects the response they receive by thinking of specific incidents you have experienced.

a. Consider incidents in which you did not receive the type of response you would have appreciated and reflect on how you felt when you made the approach and your behaviour. Jot down the behaviours you recognize.
b. Consider an incident in which someone's approach to you resulted in your responding less than positively. Jot down the behaviours you observed.

____

____

____

3. Share group members' thoughts and lists of behaviours that contribute to less than positive responses.

____

____

____

4. Consolidate the behaviours identified, list on your flip chart and be prepared to share it with the larger group.

____

____

____

WORKOUT 9: IT'S YOUR CHOICE

Element strengthened: *Change Compatibility*

Time Required: 35 minutes to 2.5 hours

- Activity 1: 35 minutes
- Activity 2: 45 minutes
- Activity 3: 1 hour

Note: The three activities can be presented together for a 2.5-hour workshop, or they can be presented individually.

Objective

To strengthen the change compatibility element by:

- Recognizing how an individual's attitude and thoughts directly impact his or her response to change
- Learning how to replace negative thoughts with more productive ones so as to change individual and team responses to change

Background

The dictionary defines *attitude* as "a way of looking at life; a way of thinking, feeling or behaving."[1]

Attitude is made up of thoughts, feelings, and behaviours, and each of these three things has a direct impact on the results we create in our life and work. The good news is that every individual has the power to choose his or her own thoughts and behaviours.

High-performing teams are experts at practicing the art of mindfulness. They are aware of their thinking patterns and how their thoughts impact the way they feel and behave. They know that their thoughts have a direct impact on the results they create. High-performing teams and individuals know that it is not what happens to them in life that creates their experience, but how they respond to what happens. They can therefore create more positive experiences by choosing productive thoughts and behaviours.

Being mindful of our response is especially important when dealing with change. This is particularly true when people are fearful of or are not supportive of a change. Fear and lack of support will often result in negative thoughts, feelings, and behaviour, which can hamper the successful implementation of the change, as well as create increased stress for those involved. An essential coping and change-management strategy is to recognize the thoughts and feelings being created in response to a stressful situation, and to consciously choose to replace the unproductive thoughts with productive ones that will result in a more positive experience.

Materials Required

- PowerPoint slide: ItsAllAboutAttitude.ppt found at www.healthcareteamperformance.com
- Handouts (listed below), which are included here and can also be found at www.healthcareteamperformance.com

Activity 1 Handout

- You Have the Power to Choose

Activity 2 Handout

- The Power of Thought

Activity 3 Handouts

- A Model for Managing Change and Stress
- Managing Change and Stress
- My Commitments to Action

Preparation

- Complete the following activities/handouts so that you have a solid understanding of what the participants will experience in this workshop.
  - You Have the Power to Choose
  - The Power of Thought

  Note: You might choose to customize the examples on "The Power of Thought" handout to reflect situations experienced in your participants' work environment.
- Review the handout "A Model for Managing Change and Stress" to ensure you have a clear understanding of the information you will be sharing.
- Complete the handout "Managing Change and Stress."

Activity 1

Time Required: 35 minutes

Steps

1. Show the quote on slide 1 ("It's not what happens to us in life that creates our experience, but how we respond to what happens") and generate a discussion (10 minutes). You might use the following to help you do so:

   ASK What does this quote mean to you?

   COMMON RESPONSES

   - You can choose a variety of responses to any given situation.
   - We tend to blame the situation for how we feel instead of looking at our own response to it.
   - We have complete control over how we respond to any situation and therefore have control over what we experience in life.

   ASK How does this quote apply to managing change?

   COMMON RESPONSES

   - Even if we don't agree with the change, we will make the situation worse by focusing only on the negative.
   - If we change our response we can change our experience.
   - If we respond more positively we will have a more positive experience.

2. Share information from the Objective and Background sections of this workout. You might say:

SAY Our objective for today is to improve our ability to manage change by learning to choose our responses to situations involving change.

SHARE THE FOLLOWING

We often don't think about choosing a response; we just react. The good news is that we do have the power to choose our behaviour and our thoughts. High-performing teams are experts at practising the art of mindfulness. They are aware of their thinking patterns and how their thoughts impact the way they feel and behave. They know that their thoughts have a direct impact on the results they create. High-performing teams and individuals know that it is not what happens to them in life that creates their experience, but how they respond to what happens. They can therefore create positive experiences by *choosing* productive thoughts and behaviours. And so can we.

Being mindful of our response is especially important when dealing with change. This is particularly true when people are fearful of or are not supportive of a change. Fear and lack of support will often result in negative thoughts, feelings, and behaviour, which can hamper the successful implementation of the change, as well as create increased stress for those involved. An essential coping and change-management strategy is to recognize the thoughts and feelings being created in response to a stressful situation, and then consciously choose to replace the unproductive thoughts with more productive ones that will result in a more positive experience.

Show slide 2.

3. Distribute the handout "You Have the Power to Choose." Allow 10 minutes for completion.
4. Ask members to share their observations/thoughts with a partner.
5. Give members the opportunity to share any observations/thoughts with the larger group, should they choose to do so.
6. Ask each member to make a personal commitment to being aware of his or her response when a change situation arises and to choosing a positive response.

Activity 2

Time Required: 45 minutes

Steps

1. Share the following objective of this activity: to learn to adjust our response to change by replacing negative thoughts with positive ones.

> **SAY** Let's talk about the power of thoughts for a minute. Researchers have determined that the average person—that means you—talks to themselves 50,000 times a day. Fifty thousand times a day! Now, some of you are thinking, "What is she talking about? I don't talk to myself, she's crazy." But you do talk to yourself—50,000 times a day, in fact. And the most astonishing part of this statistic is that 80 per cent of the time our self-talk is negative—80 per cent of the time we are thinking negatively about ourselves, about another person, or about a situation, event, work environment, etc. So if we have negative thoughts 80 per cent of the time, how are we feeling 80 per cent of the time?
>
> *Negative*, that's right. And when we are stressed, tired, and overwhelmed, there is more conflict and we display more negative behaviours.
>
> We also know from research that these thoughts have a powerful effect on us. They affect our attitude, our physiology, and our motivation to act. Our negative thoughts actually control our behaviour.

2. Ask individuals to pick up all of their belongings and change seats so that they are sitting with new people. Tell them they have 15 seconds. Note: The purpose of this is to have participants experience a sudden, unexpected change.

> **ASK** How did it feel to suddenly change?

ASK What might make some people uncomfortable about this change and how we went about it?

COMMON RESPONSES

- No structure, no real plan as to how to change seats.
- Not sure why we were changing seats.
- Not knowing who we would be working with, what working with them would be like.
- We were comfortable the way we were.

ASK What is the lesson here? What was the purpose of this exercise?

ASK How can we apply this learning to managing change?

SHARE THE FOLLOWING

Every change involves some form of loss and letting go of something that is familiar. The status quo, by definition, is the existing way of doing things. It is the way things already are, and for that reason it can be attractive. But the status quo has to change, especially in the incredibly fast-paced, ever-evolving world we live in. If we don't keep changing and striving to be better, then mediocrity and complacency set in.

Change is often feared because it involves moving away from our comfort zone. Our comfort zone is stress free; there are very few unknowns, if any; it is predictable. But there is no growth in the comfort zone. Growth happens when we step outside of it and start trying new things and taking risks with the intent to improve ourselves. But moving from our comfort zone requires going from the known to the unknown—and this can create anxiety and stress, which can lead to greater conflict and negatively impact teamwork as a result.

(*continued*)

> Change, as you all know, is a sure constant in life; therefore, it is essential to be prepared for change and to be prepared to step outside of your comfort zone, because change often happens when we least expect it. And by being prepared, I mean taking the time to reflect on how you respond to change, and identifying ways to ensure you respond in a manner that will help you thrive in times of change. Then, when change does occur, you will be able to choose to respond in a manner that will create a positive experience and positive results.

3. Distribute the handout "The Power of Thought, Part A" and share the following:

> **SAY** You're going to experience the power of thought with this first exercise. You'll see a number of situations outlined on your handout; choose three that would create stress or a negative thought for you. For each situation, I want you to put yourself right into the situation by imagining exactly what it would be like. Picture it in your mind, see what you see, hear what you hear, and feel what you feel. Then write down any negative thoughts that come to mind in the situation. Next, write down what you experience as a result. Do you feel frustrated or insecure? How would you behave if you were acting out the situation? What might the result be?
>
> Take 10 minutes.

4. Debrief. Ask for participants to share their examples.
5. Distribute "The Power of Thought, Part B" and share the following:

> **SAY** For each of the situations you chose in the first part, identify a new thought—a more positive thought that will replace the negative one. Then identify the results you would experience.
>
> Take 10 minutes.

6. Ask each member to describe a lesson to take away from the exercise.

Activity 3

Time Required: 1 hour

Steps

1. Distribute the handout "A Model for Managing Change and Stress" and review with the group. Refer to slide 3.
2. Distribute the "Managing Change and Stress" handout and allow 20 minutes for participants to complete and to share with a partner.
3. Debrief. Ask individuals to share their examples.
4. Distribute the "My Commitments to Action" handout and allow five minutes to complete.
5. Ask individuals to share their commitments to action and any "ah-ha" moments or key learnings they gained from the session.

Handout
Page 1 of 2

POWER OF THOUGHT

Part A

Situation	Trigger Thought	Behaviour/Result
A patient aggressively complains about the service she/he is receiving.		
You ask a team member a question and she/he responds in an abrupt and impatient manner.		
Your team priorities change again unexpectedly.		
In front of others, a team member points out a mistake you made.		
Your manager gives you another task to complete this week (in addition to your other priorities).		
Other:		

Handout
Page 2 of 2

POWER OF THOUGHT

Part B

Situation	Trigger Thought	Behaviour/Result
A patient aggressively complains about the service she/he is receiving.		
You ask a team member a question and she/he responds in an abrupt and impatient manner.		
Your team priorities change again unexpectedly.		
In front of others, a team member points out a mistake you made.		
Your manager gives you another task to complete this week (in addition to your other priorities).		
Other:		

Handout
Page 1 of 1

YOU HAVE THE POWER TO CHOOSE!

It's not what happens to us in life that creates our experience, but how we respond to what happens.

What scares you most about change?

____

____

____

____

List examples of change at work that result in stress.

____

____

____

____

How do you respond to these situations now?

____

____

____

____

If you could choose a different, more productive and positive response to change, what would that look and feel like?

____

____

____

____

What do you stand to gain by choosing a new response?

____

____

____

____

Handout
Page 1 of 2

A MODEL FOR MANAGING CHANGE AND STRESS

By changing the way that you think about things, you are able to change the way that you feel about them.

By identifying and modifying thoughts that produce negative feelings, you are then able to improve personal and work situations and reach your goals with less stress.

A = Activating event (what happened)

An occurrence that triggers an emotional consequence.

Example:

- My bus is running late, I won't make it in time for work.
- My manager just changed my priorities again.

B = Belief (what you are thinking, self-talk)

An evaluation and judgment about the demands of yourself, demands of others, and demands of the world or life conditions. These may be rational and realistic or irrational.

Example:

- People will think badly of me for being late. They will think I'm irresponsible and unreliable.
- My manager doesn't care about my workload and how much stress I'm under.

C = Consequence (outcome)

An emotional and/or physical consequence linked to a belief.

Example:

- Anxiety.
- Frustration, rolling of the eyes, sighing, and complaining.

Handout
Page 2 of 2

MANAGING CHANGE AND STRESS

Now apply the steps from "A Model for Managing Change and Stress" to a real example from your own life.

Step 1: Think of an activating event (A)

____

____

____

____

____

____

Step 2: Identify beliefs (B) that lead to negative outcomes

____

____

____

____

____

____

Step 3: Identify your feelings/reactions (C)

____

____

____

____

____

____

Step 4: Identify how you would like to feel and behave the next time the same event occurs (Goal)

____

____

____

____

____

Handout
Page 1 of 1

MY COMMITMENTS TO ACTION

In order to better manage change, I will...

____

____

____

____

____

____

____

____

____

____

____

____

____

____

In order to help my team members better manage change, I will...

____

____

____

____

____

____

____

____

____

____

____

____

____

____

WORKOUT 10: TRUTHS FOR CHANGE

Element strengthened: *Change Compatibility*

Time Required: *1.5 to 2.5 hours (depending on anticipated depth of discussion)*

Objective

To strengthen the change compatibility element by understanding basic change-management truths related to the effective implementation of change.

Background

Although change has become increasingly complex, the effective implementation of change still depends on some basic change-management truths:

- People who plan the battle don't battle the plan. The more opportunities team members have to participate productively in a change process, the more readily they will embrace a change.
- Information is power. It is essential to share information readily and openly during a change process. If information is not available, the gap will be filled with rumors, which are often negative.
- Feeling out of control is a major cause of stress. Sharing information with team members and encouraging them to participate in the change will increase their sense of control. Stress can lead team members to more actively resist change as a defense mechanism, which can negatively affect performance.
- Stay agents are as important as change agents. Once a change is implemented, those implementing the change turn their attention to new things. Often the people who implement change do not give sufficient attention to ensuring that the change has effectively "taken." Leaders should ask: "Is it working?" "Are people adjusting well?" etc.

Note: This activity works best if the discussion can be applied to a recent change that has already been implemented, or that is in the process of being implemented. However, if an appropriate change example is not available, a discussion can be applied more generically. For example, ask, "When implementing change, how do you usually...?"

Materials Required

- Handout: "Truths For Change," which is included here and can also be found at www.healthcareteamperformance.com

Steps

1. Using the descriptions in the Background section of this workout, discuss each change truth.
2. Identify a recent change and ask team members to first assess it on their own using the handout, and then to move into discussion groups to share and build on their observations.
3. Invite each group to recap their discussion and share key points for each truth.
4. List the *growth opportunities* (GOs) identified, and develop corresponding commitments to action. For example, "We agree to..."
5. Check for consensus on the agreements, and identify methods the team can use to ensure follow through on the commitments.

Handout
Page 1 of 2

TRUTHS FOR CHANGE

1. Discuss how each of these management truths applies to change within this team.
2. Identify examples of how each truth was or was not followed, and list anything the team would benefit from doing differently.

People who plan the battle don't battle the plan.

Actions or behaviours that have supported this truth:

____

____

____

Actions or behaviours that have ignored this truth:

____

____

____

GOs (growth opportunities/what we need to do differently):

____

____

____

Information is power.

Actions or behaviours that have supported this truth:

____

____

____

Actions or behaviours that have ignored this truth:

____

____

____

Handout
Page 1 of 2

GOs (growth opportunities/what we need to do differently):

____

____

____

Feeling out of control is a major cause of stress.

Actions or behaviours that have supported this truth:

____

____

____

Actions or behaviours that have ignored this truth:

____

____

____

GOs (growth opportunities/what we need to do differently):

____

____

____

Stay agents are as important as change agents.

Actions or behaviours that have supported this truth:

____

____

____

Actions or behaviours that have ignored this truth:

____

____

____

GOs (growth opportunities/what we need to do differently):

____

____

____

WORKOUT 11: AS OTHERS SEE US

Element strengthened: *Team Members' Contribution*

Time Required: *45 minutes or more*

Objective

To strengthen the team members' contribution element by challenging team members to reflect on their personal style and make commitments to strengthening their personal contribution to the team.

Background

Growth happens when individuals pause to reflect on their performance or behaviour, identify strengths and opportunities for growth, and act on these opportunities. Before moving into the activity, spend a little time discussing this and preparing team members to receive input from their colleagues.

Important Note: This activity can be extremely beneficial in moving the team forward. However, because this activity asks that members' behaviours be addressed, sensitive issues could arise. Following the instructions carefully is important, as they are designed to manage the process effectively. However, should you anticipate any serious issues, ensure that the individual facilitating the activity has sufficient experience to make this is a comfortable and rewarding experience for everyone.

Materials Required

- Handout: "As Others See Us," included here and can also be found at www.healthcareteamperformance.com

Steps

1. Tell the group that this activity is designed to support each team member in tapping the best of him or herself and becoming an even stronger team member. You might add that in our busy workdays, we seldom take time

to reflect on what we are doing well and how we could improve ourselves. This activity provides that opportunity.

2. Distribute copies of the participants' worksheet "As Others See Us" to each member.
3. Ask the group to break into pairs.
4. Explain that each person is to complete two "As Others See Us" worksheets, one for themselves and one for their partner. They then compare the strengths they have identified in themselves to the ones their partner has identified for them. After comparing their assessments, ask each person to consider the characteristics they did not check off as their strengths, and identify at least one area that they will work on improving.
5. Allow approximately 25 minutes for the partners to complete the worksheets and discuss them. (If there are particular issues that are likely to be brought out in the discussion, more time may be required.)
6. Ask each member to share a characteristic that both members of the pair identified as a strength for that member, plus one opportunity for growth (a characteristic or behaviour that is not seen as a strength).

   Tip: It works well to have the partner talk about strengths that the member brings to the team, and to have the member being discussed identify his or her own opportunities for personal growth.
7. Invite members to make commitments to action for strengthening their opportunities for growth.

Handout
Page 1 of 2

AS OTHERS SEE US

Consider the characteristics below and put an X beside those that describe *you.*

____ Co-operative	____ Willing to compromise
____ Informed	____ Copes well with change
____ Participative	____ Follows through on commitments
____ Organized	____ Examines issues objectively
____ Trustworthy	____ Resistant to change
____ Positive (approaches issues constructively)	____ Judges quickly
____ Negative (tends to look for the problems, not the solutions)	____ Highly skilled in job/ profession
____ Open and honest	____ High personal work standards
____ Aggressive	____ Can be depended on
____ Assertive	____ Reluctant to move from one position or point of view
____ A natural leader	____ Makes others feel good about themselves
____ Easy to deal with	____ Flexible
____ Often involved in conflict	____ Sees others' points of view
____ The one who resolves conflict	

Handout
Page 2 of 2

AS OTHERS SEE US

Consider the same characteristics and put an X beside those that describe *your partner.*

____ Co-operative	____ Willing to compromise
____ Informed	____ Copes well with change
____ Participative	____ Follows through on commitments
____ Organized	____ Examines issues objectively
____ Trustworthy	____ Resistant to change
____ Positive (approaches issues constructively)	____ Judges quickly
____ Negative (tends to look for the problems, not the solutions)	____ Highly skilled in job/ profession
____ **Open and honest**	____ High personal work standards
____ Aggressive	____ Can be depended on
____ Assertive	____ Reluctant to move from one position or point of view
____ A natural leader	____ Makes others feel good about themselves
____ Easy to deal with	____ Flexible
____ Often involved in conflict	____ Sees others' points of view
____ The one who resolves conflict	

WORKOUT 12: WE'RE ALL RESPONSIBLE

Element strengthened: *Team Members' Contribution*

Time Required: *45 minutes to 1 hour*

Objective

To strengthen the team members' contribution element by increasing the team's sense of responsibility for identifying opportunities to improve care practice/service delivery.

Background

It is unlikely that team members will look for opportunities to improve care practice/service delivery unless they perceive that it is their responsibility and part of their job. This activity is designed to remind members that improvement is indeed their responsibility, and it will put that responsibility in the forefront of their minds.

Materials Required

None

Preparation

Ask members to come to the session prepared to share at least one idea for improving care practice/service delivery in their team.

Steps

1. Ask members to share the ideas they brought to the session.
2. Discuss as many ideas as time allows, and congratulate members on the ideas they have generated.
3. Help the team to devise a plan for taking the ideas forward and ensuring they are implemented.
4. Ask members why they don't automatically bring forward good ideas like the ones they brought to this session. Answers may include the following:
   - We are too busy.
   - We don't see this as part of our job.
   - We don't think that our recommendations will be used.
5. Discuss the points generated. Facilitate consensus for one or two commitments to action in order to improve care practice/service delivery.

WORKOUT 13: THE COLOUR OF INFLUENCE

Element strengthened:* *Shared Leadership

Time Required: *30 minutes to 1 hour or more (depending on depth of discussion)*

Objective

To strengthen the shared leadership element by determining the degree to which team members feel they have influence/power within the team and by clarifying perceptions of influence.

Background

A sense of shared leadership and influence are key to high-performance teams. If members feel they have little influence, it is unlikely they will feel a sense of ownership for the success of the team.

This workout asks members to consider the degree to which they feel they have influence within the team. If influence is seen as unbalanced, the team explores why, and determines how a greater equalization of voices can be achieved.

Note: If team members do not feel they have power, it may be due to the leader's style and the leader must be open to exploring this possibility.

Materials Required

- Red, green, blue, and yellow paper squares or circles, about 2" × 2" (50 cm × 50 cm); one of each colour for each participant
- Two envelopes for each participant, one containing the coloured squares, and one labelled "Response" (ensure colours cannot be easily seen through the envelope)

Steps

1. Distribute the envelopes.
2. Explain to the participants that in one envelope they will find four coloured squares: one red, one green, one blue, and one yellow. Ask them to consider the degree to which they feel they have influence within the team, and to select a coloured square according to the following:

Red—I have a great deal of influence
Green—I have quite a bit of influence
Blue—I have little influence
Yellow—I have no influence

Put the above on a flip chart, board, or slide. Give participants sufficient time to seriously consider their response.

Note: Ensure that participants are seated far enough apart to be able to select a colour privately. Ask participants to put the coloured square they select into the envelope labelled "Response."

3. Collect the Response envelopes.
4. Ask the participants what they considered when determining their degree of influence. Record responses on a board, flip chart, or slide.

COMMON RESPONSES

- It depends on whether my opinion is asked.
- It depends on whether my ideas are listened to.
- It depends on whether outcomes are influenced by my input.

5. Display the squares on a board or flip chart, putting like colours close together.
6. Describe the pattern suggested. For example, "Most people feel they have a good deal of influence, but a few feel they have little influence."

ASK Why might this be the case?

ASK How does this affect team outcomes?

ASK Does this pattern and/or discussion suggest anything that we as a team or as individuals should be doing differently?

Capture responses on the flip chart.

COMMON RESPONSES

- We need to speak up more.
- We need to listen more effectively to one another.
- We need to invite each other's input more often.
- We need to more carefully consider who should be involved in a decision.

7. Identify at least two commitments to action (behaviours or practices that team members will change) that the team agrees to live by in order to create greater shared leadership.
8. Discuss and identify how team members will keep one another accountable for their commitments. For example, agree to review commitments to action at least once a month to keep on track.
9. Recap outcomes and thank the team for its participation.

WORKOUT 14: TOWARD INCREASED SELF-DIRECTION

Element strengthened: *Shared Leadership*

Time Required: *45 minutes to 1 hour*

Objective

To strengthen the shared leadership element by increasing the team's level of self-direction (empowerment) and by establishing increased participation and self-direction as a team development goal.

Background

When teams share leadership, they have an appropriate degree of self-direction. This may differ from task to task, and will change as the team develops. Your team's degree of self-direction can be determined using the Levels of Influence figure that is illustrated below.

A team leader could define his or her primary responsibility as the continuous development of the team toward increased self-direction.

Note: This activity is effective only if the team leader is ready, willing, and able to let go and further empower team members.

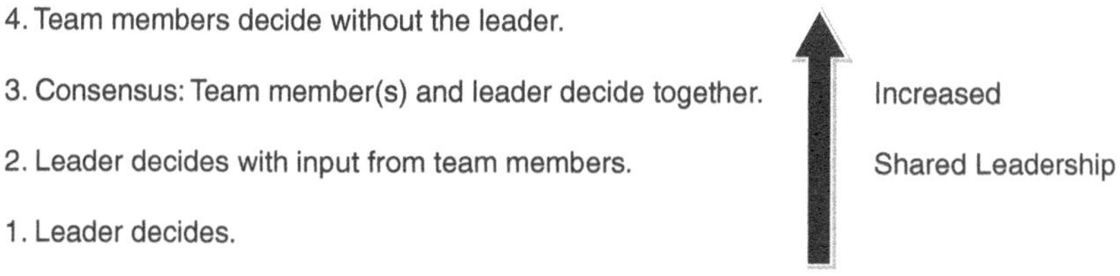

4. Team members decide without the leader.

3. Consensus: Team member(s) and leader decide together.

2. Leader decides with input from team members.

1. Leader decides.

↑ Increased Shared Leadership

Figure 13.1: Levels of Influence

Materials Required

- Handout: "Levels of Influence" which is included here and can also be found at www.healthcareteamperformance.com

Steps

1. Introduce team members to the Levels of Influence using the information provided in the Background section of this workout.

2. Distribute the "Levels of Influence" handout. Allow 10 minutes for its completion.
3. Ask team members to share their observations, and from these ideas develop a list of decisions made at a level 1 or 2 that could have benefited from being made at a 3 or 4.
4. Recap the discussion and check for consensus on any commitments to action made.

ASK What benefits would be reaped by moving these types of decisions to a higher level?

ASK What do you need to do to ensure that the team increases the frequency with which it works at the higher levels?

COMMON RESPONSES

- We must continue to develop skills to enable us to function effectively at higher levels of influence.
- When we see an opportunity to function at a higher level, we must bring it to the leader's and the team's attention.
- We must be willing to take the responsibility and accountability that go with increased empowerment.

Handout
Page 1 of 1

LEVELS OF INFLUENCE

Allotted time: 10 minutes

Identify a decision that was recently made in your team at a 1 or 2 level that would have benefited from a level 3 or 4 process. Jot down ways in which the team would have benefited.

Decision:

____
____
____
____
____

Level at which the decision was made:

____
____
____
____
____

Level at which we recommend the decision be made in the future:

____
____
____
____
____

Ways in which the team will benefit from decision making at this level:

____
____
____
____
____

WORKOUT 15: NEVER WASTE A MISTAKE

Element strengthened: *Shared Learning*

Time Required: *25 minutes to 1 hour*

Objective

To help ensure that mistakes lead to learning.

Background

Every error or event provides an important learning opportunity. That learning does not happen if blame is present, if feedback is poorly given, or if an opportunity to learn from the error is not provided.

Materials Required:

- Flip chart

Steps

1. Write the following statement on a flip chart or white board:

   Never waste a mistake.

2. Generate discussion with the following:

ASK	How do we waste mistakes?

COMMON RESPONSES

- By not learning from them.
- By ignoring them.
- By spending time blaming.

Capture responses on the flip chart.

ASK What behaviours and practices need to be present to ensure there is an opportunity to learn from mistakes?

COMMON RESPONSES

- We need to focus on the incident, not the individual.
- We need to give feedback effectively so that the individual and others can hear and apply the learning.
- We need to be receptive to input.
- We need to take time to fully discuss important incidents.
- We need to follow up on discussion to ensure appropriate practices are implemented.

3. Check for agreement on the ideas.
4. Turn the agreed upon items into commitments to action.
5. Facilitate an agreement on a method for keeping the commitments alive.

WORKOUT 16: LEARNING FROM EACH OTHER

Element strengthened: *Shared Learning*

Time Required: *35 minutes*

Objective

To strengthen the shared learning element by:

- Reinforcing the importance of sharing knowledge and experience
- Helping team members to recognize previously overlooked opportunities to share learning.

Materials Required

- Flip chart

Steps

1. Generate a discussion:

ASK What benefits of shared learning have you experienced or observed?

COMMON RESPONSES

- We can't all have learned everything on our own. Sharing multiplies the knowledge in the team.
- By sharing our experience from errors or near misses, we can support one another in preventing future incidents.
- Readily sharing learning with one another builds a sense of team.
- We learn more about and better appreciate each other's experience and knowledge.

COMMON RESPONSES

- We are too busy to think about sharing.
- Sometimes people feel like their knowledge is their power and if they share it they will lose power.
- We don't always know what would be useful to someone else.

2. Think of an instance when you a) could have learned from someone else and b) could have shared your learning with someone. For each example consider why the learning opportunity was not seized. From these observations develop at least two recommendations for ensuring that shared learning opportunities are not missed in the future.

   Note: This step can be performed individually or in small groups.
3. Invite individuals or groups to share their examples and reasons as to why the opportunities were missed.
4. Invite individuals or groups to share their two recommendations.
5. Turn the recommendations into commitments to action as appropriate.

ENERGIZE YOUR MEETINGS WITH BRAINTEASERS

Highly effective meetings, whether they are team meetings or team development sessions, are ones in which team members are focused, participating in team dialogue, and generating innovative ideas and solutions.

An effective way to energize your team and ensure productive participation is to introduce brainteasers at the beginning of your meeting. Introducing brainteasers can help you succeed in one or all of the following:

- Getting people's heads in the meeting. When they enter the meeting room, team members are often preoccupied with the work they have left behind. Focusing on brainteasers forces them to set everything else aside.
- Sparking creative thinking. We ask our team members to be creative, and to think outside the box, but often we provide them with only a "boxlike" meeting and thinking environment. For example, we hold meetings in the same room, we sit in the same place at the meeting table, we stick to a predictable agenda, or we maintain the same tone or atmosphere.

  Brainteasers change the tone of the meeting, which in itself encourages different thinking. In addition, brainteasers demand that participants exercise a part of their brain that usually isn't tapped during traditional problem-solving sessions. Studies have shown that innovation is much more likely to emerge in an environment in which people are having fun.
- Increasing participation. Brainteasers warm the group up. Participants generally find it easy and fun to take part in a brainteaser activity. When they discover that participating is non-threatening, and even enjoyable, they tend to continue in a heightened participatory mode once the team moves on to the meeting agenda.

If the meeting has a team-building element, then there is an additional benefit to encouraging members to solve a set of brainteasers together as a team. The advantages of working as a team will quickly become apparent as each member brings his or her own particular perceptions, skills, and experience to the puzzle-solving process.

TIP

Breaking the group into smaller teams to solve the brainteasers, and pitting the teams against one another, can add an additional element of fun. It also encourages people to move into a "working together" mode.

BRAINTEASER #1
Something in Common

Clue
Napkin
Nose
Circus

Answer
Ring

What do each of these words have in common?

1. Floor
   Car
   Candle

2. Brief
   Camera
   Cosmetic

3. Paper
   Report
   Stand

4. Record
   Clock
   Example

5. Sign
   Watch
   Gap

6. Post
   Stop
   Astrological

BRAINTEASER #2

Tease Your Brain!

Clue
BLFLOWERSOOM

Answer
Flowers in bloom

Find the expression or phrase that each of these represents:

1. SOME
SOME

2. PERFORMANCE
PERFORMANCE

3. N
O
S
E

4. BAN ANA

5. **D
R
A
F
T**

6. KOOL

7. S
E
C
SECTION
I
O
N

8. WEATHER
FEELING

BRAINTEASER #3

Tease Your Brain!

Clue

BLFLOWERSOOM

Answer

Flowers in bloom

Find the expression or phrase that each of these represents:

1. WOMEN
   HE
2. MIH TO THE
   LAW
3. SAIL SAIL
4. LINEREADLINE
5. BELIEF IT
6. JOBHEJOB

BRAINTEASER #4

Tease Your Brain!

Clue

BLFLOWERSOOM

Answer

Flowers in bloom

Find the expression or phrase that each of these represents:

1. LOVE SIGHT
   SIGHT
   SIGHT

2. ALL
   BOARD

3. CRJEWELOWN

4. C
   O
   U
   N
   T

5. EVENTS

6. VIEW

7. TUNNEL LIGHT

8. PEAK PEAK

BRAINTEASER #5

Something in Common

Clue
Napkin
Nose
Circus

Answer
Ring

What do each of these words have in common?

1. Strap
   Boot
   Case

2. Door
   Cow
   School

3. Fast
   Junk
   Gourmet

4. Brass
   Tree
   Mountain

5. Button
   Cart
   Over

6. Soup
   Gun
   Face

7. Flakes
   Fall
   Ball

8. Hockey
   Broom
   Gum

ANSWERS TO BRAINTEASERS

Brainteaser #1

1. The word *wax*
2. They are types of cases
3. News can describe each
4. They can be set
5. Stop can describe each
6. The word *sign*

Brainteaser #2

1. Twosome
2. Repeat performance
3. Nosedive
4. Banana split
5. Downward draft
6. Look backwards
7. Cross-section
8. Feeling under the weather

Brainteaser #3

1. He's after women
2. Turn him over to the law
3. Parasail
4. Read between the lines
5. It's beyond belief
6. He's between jobs

Brainteaser #4

1. Love at first sight
2. All above board
3. Jewel in the crown
4. Countdown
5. Turn of events
6. Slanted view
7. Light at the end of the tunnel
8. Twin peaks

Brainteaser #5

1. They can be made of leather
2. They are types of bells
3. They are types of food
4. The word *top*
5. The word *push* precedes each
6. The word *powder* can follow each
7. The word *snow* precedes each
8. They are types of sticks

Endnotes

INTRODUCTION

1. A. M. Rafferty et al., "Are Teamwork and Professional Autonomy Compatible, and Do They Result in Improved Hospital Care?" *Quality in Health Care* 10, suppl. 2 (December 2001): ii32–ii37.
2. K. Keutner et al., "Nurses Job Satisfaction and Organizational Climate in a Dynamic Work Environment," *Applied Nursing Research* 13, no. 1 (2000): 46–49; S. Kangas, C. Kee, and R. McKee-Waddle, "Organization Factors, Nurses' Job Satisfaction, and Patient Satisfaction with Nursing Care," *Journal of Nursing Administration* 29, no. 1 (1999): 32–42; H. Tzeng, S. Ketefian, and R. Redman, "Relationship of Nurses' Assessment of Organizational Culture, Job Satisfaction, and Patient Satisfaction within Nursing Care," *International Journal of Nursing Studies* 39, no. 1 (2002): 79–84.
3. Donald C. Cole et al., "Quality of Working Life Indicators in Canadian Health Care Organizations: A Tool for Healthy, Healthcare Workplaces." *Occupational Medicine* 55, (2005): 54–59.
4. C. L. Stavins, "Developing Employee Participation in the Patient Satisfaction Process," ACHE: Fellowship Case Reports (2006). Retrieved September 5, 2006, from http://www.ache.org/mbership/AdvtoFellow/CASERPTS/stavins02.cfm

CHAPTER 1

1. Michael Kent, *The Oxford Dictionary of Sports Science & Medicine*, s.v. "team dynamics" (Oxford University Press, 2006).

CHAPTER 2

1. K. Keutner et al., "Nurses Job Satisfaction and Organizational Climate in a Dynamic Work Environment," *Applied Nursing Research* 13,

no. 1 (2000): 46–49; S. Kangas, C. Kee, and R. McKee-Waddle, "Organization Factors, Nurses' Job Satisfaction, and Patient Satisfaction with Nursing Care," *Journal of Nursing Administration* 29, no. 1 (1999): 32–42; H. Tzeng, S. Ketefian, and R. Redman, "Relationship of Nurses' Assessment of Organizational Culture, Job Satisfaction, and Patient Satisfaction within Nursing Care," *International Journal of Nursing Studies* 39, no. 1 (2002): 79–84.

2. Robert Shaw, *Trust in the Balance: Building Successful Organizations on Results, Integrity and Concern* (San Francisco: Jossey-Bass Inc., 1997).
3. H. K. S. Laschinger, "Hospital Nurses' Perceptions of Respect and Organizational Justice," *Journal of Nursing Administration* 34 (2004): 354–64.
4. H. K. S. Laschinger, "Building Healthy Workplaces: Time to Act on the Evidence," *Healthcare Papers* 7, Special Issue (2007): 42–45.
5. L. Sofield, "Workplace Violence: A Focus on Verbal Abuse and Intent to Leave the Organization," *Orthopaedic Nursing* 22, no. 4 (July/August 2003): 274–83.
6. J. E. Boychuk Duchscher, "Out in the Real World: Newly Graduate Nurses in Acute-Care Speak Out," *Journal of Nursing Administration* 31, no. 9 (September 2001): 426–39.
7. C. Garcia Vivar, "Putting Conflict Management into Practice: A Nursing Case Study," *Journal of Nursing Management* 14, no. 3 (April 2006): 201–06.
8. Leslie Bendaly, *Leadership on the Run: How to Get Better Results Faster* (Toronto: Viking Canada, 2004).

CHAPTER 3

1. A. J. Ducanis and A. K. Golin, *The Interdisciplinary Health Care Team: A Handbook* (Germantown, MD: Aspen Publishers, 1979).
2. Janet Davidson, in discussion with Nicole Bendaly, February 9, 2012.
3. Institute of Medicine: Committee on Quality of Health Care in America, *Crossing the Quality Chasm: A New Health System for the 21st Century* (Washington, DC: National Academies Press, 2001).
4. Ibid.
5. J. Carpenter et al., "Working in Multidisciplinary Community Mental Health Teams: The Impact on Social Workers and Health Professionals

of Integrated Mental Health Care," *British Journal of Social Work* 33, no. 8 (2003): 1081–1103.

6. T. F. Lyons, "Role Clarity, Need for Clarity, Satisfaction, Tension, and Withdrawal," *Organizational Behavior and Human Performance* 6 (1971): 99–110.
7. C. Mariano, "The Case for Interdisciplinary Collaboration," *Nursing Outlook* (November/December 1989): 286–89.
8. Lyons, "Role Clarity," 99–110.
9. C. A. Orchard, V. Curran, S. Kabene, "Creating a Culture for Interdisciplinary Collaborative Professional Practice," *Medical Education Online* (serial online) 10 (2005): 11.
10. Leonard Berry and Kent Seltman, *Management Lessons from Mayo Clinic: Inside one of the World's Most Admired Service Organizations* (New York: McGraw-Hill, 2008).
11. T. Butler and J. Waldroop, "Job Sculpting, the Art of Retaining your Best People," *Harvard Business Review* (September 1999). http://hbr.org/1999/09/job-sculpting-the-art-of-retaining-your-best-people/ar/1

CHAPTER 4

1. S. G. Kirby, "Communication Among Healthcare Professionals: An Essential Component of Quality Care," North Carolina Medical Board Newsletter no. 4 (2010).
2. K. Sutcliffe et al., "Communication Failures: An Insidious Contributor to Medical Errors," *Journal of Academic Medicine* 70, no. 2 (2004): 186–94.
3. Leslie Bendaly, *Leadership on the Run: How to Get Better Results Faster* (Toronto: Viking Canada, 2004).
4. D. Laws and S. Amato, "Incorporating Bedside Reporting into Change-of-Shift Report," *Rehabilitation Nursing* 35, no. 2 (March/April 2010): 70–74.

CHAPTER 5

1. Rosabeth Moss Kanter, *The Change Masters* (New York: Simon and Schuster, 1984).

CHAPTER 8

1. Peter Senge, *The Fifth Discipline: The Art & Practice of the Learning Organization,* (New York: Doubleday, 2006), 9.
2. National Health Service Management Executive, *Nursing in Primary Care—New World, New Opportunities* (Leeds: NHSME, 1993).
3. Bruce Harber and Ted Hall, "From Blame Game to Accountability in Healthcare," *Policy Options/Options Politiques* (November 2003): 49–54.
4. Heather Childers, "FAA Sees Surge in Reports of Air-Traffic Errors," *FoxNews.com,* February 25, 2011.
5. Ibid.
6. Institute of Medicine: Committee on Quality of Health Care in America, *Crossing the Quality Chasm: A New Health System for the 21st Century* (Washington, DC: National Academies Press, 2001), 79.
7. A. C. Edmonson, "Learning from Failure in Health Care: Frequent Opportunities, Pervasive Barriers," *Quality and Safety in Healthcare* 13, suppl. 2 (2004): ii3–ii9.

CHAPTER 12

1. Leslie Bendaly, *On Track: Taking Meetings from Good to Great* (Toronto: McGraw-Hill Ryerson, 2002).

Bibliography

Bendaly, Leslie. *Leadership on the Run: How to Get Better Results Faster.* Toronto: Viking Canada, 2004.

Bendaly, Leslie. *On Track: Taking Meetings from Good to Great.* Toronto: McGraw-Hill Ryerson, 2002.

Berry, Leonard, and Kent Seltman. *Management Lessons from Mayo Clinic: Inside one of the World's Most Admired Service Organizations.* New York: McGraw-Hill, 2008.

Borrill, C. S., et al. *The Effectiveness of Healthcare Teams in the National Health Service.* Final report submitted to the Department of Health, 2000.

Boychuk Duchscher, J. E. "Out in the Real World: Newly Graduate Nurses in Acute-Care Speak Out." *Journal of Nursing Administration* 31, no. 9 (September 2001): 426–39.

Carpenter, J., et al. "Working in Multidisciplinary Community Mental Health Teams: The Impact on Social Workers and Health Professionals of Integrated Mental Health Care." *British Journal of Social Work* 33, no. 8 (2003): 1081–1103.

Childers, Heather. "FAA Sees Surge in Reports of Air-Traffic Errors." *FoxNews.com*, February 25, 2011.

Cole, Donald C., et al. "Quality of Working Life Indicators in Canadian Health Care Organizations: A Tool for Healthy, Healthcare Workplaces?" *Occupational Medicine* 55 (2005): 54–59.

Ducanis, A. J., and A. K. Golin. *The Interdisciplinary Health Care Team: A Handbook.* Germantown, MD: Aspen Publishers, 1979.

Edmonson, A. C. "Learning from Failure in Health Care: Frequent Opportunities, Pervasive Barriers." *Quality and Safety in Healthcare* 13, suppl. 2 (2004): ii3–ii9.

Garcia Vivar, C. "Putting Conflict Management into Practice: A Nursing Case Study." *Journal of Nursing Management* 14, no. 3 (April 2006): 201–06.

Harber, Bruce, and Ted Hall. "From Blame Game to Accountability in Healthcare." *Policy Options/Options Politiques* (November 2003): 49–54.

Institute of Medicine: Committee on Quality of Health Care in America. *Crossing the Quality Chasm: A New Health System for the 21st Century.* Washington, DC: National Academies Press, 2001.

Kangas, S., C. Kee, and R. McKee-Waddle. "Organization Factors, Nurses' Job Satisfaction, and Patient Satisfaction with Nursing Care." *Journal of Nursing Administration* 29, no. 1 (1999): 32–42.

Keutner, K., J. Byrne, and E. Larson. "Nurses Job Satisfaction and Organizational Climate in a Dynamic Work Environment." *Applied Nursing Research* 13, no. 1 (2000): 46–49.

Laschinger, H. K. S. "Building Healthy Workplaces: Time to Act on the Evidence." *Healthcare Papers* 7, Special Issue (2007): 42–45.

Laschinger, H. K. S. "Hospital Nurses' Perceptions of Respect and Organizational Justice." *Journal of Nursing Administration* 34 (2004): 354–64.

Laws, D., and S. Amato. "Incorporating Bedside Reporting into Change-of-Shift Report." *Rehabilitation Nursing* 35, no. 2 (March/April 2010): 70–74.

Lyons, T. F. "Role Clarity, Need for Clarity, Satisfaction, Tension, and Withdrawal." *Organizational Behavior and Human Performance* 6 (1971): 99–110.

Mariano, C. "The Case for Interdisciplinary Collaboration." *Nursing Outlook* (November/December 1989): 286–89.

Orchard, C. A., V. Curran, and S. Kabene. "Creating a Culture for Interdisciplinary Collaborative Professional Practice." *Medical Education Online* (serial online) 10 (2005): 11.

Rafferty, A. M., et al. "Are Teamwork and Professional Autonomy Compatible, and Do They Result in Improved Hospital Care?" *Quality in Health Care* 10, suppl. 2 (December 2001): ii32–ii37.

Sofield, L. "Workplace Violence: A Focus on Verbal Abuse and Intent to Leave the Organization." *Orthopaedic Nursing* 22, no. 4 (July/August 2003): 274–83.

Stavins, C.L. "Developing Employee Participation in the Patient Satisfaction Process," *Journal of Healthcare Management.* 2004 Mar–Apr; 49(2): 135–9.

Sutcliffe, K., et al. "Communication Failures: An Insidious Contributor to Medical Mishaps." *Journal of Academic Medicine* 79, no. 2 (2004): 186–94.

Tzeng, H., S. Ketefian, and R. Redman. "Relationship of Nurses' Assessment of Organizational Culture, Job Satisfaction, and Patient Satisfaction within Nursing Care." *International Journal of Nursing Studies* 39, no. 1 (2002): 79–84.

About the Authors

Leslie Bendaly is recognized as a leading thinker and practitioner in the areas of organizational leadership, teamwork, and change. She is the founder of Kinect Inc. and author of several books on leadership, including *Strength in Numbers*, *Winner Instinct*, and *Leadership on the Run*. Her models, tools, and books are used in organizations worldwide, and her books have been selected as mandatory reading for MBA and other postgraduate programs in both the U.S. and Canada.

Nicole Bendaly is president of Kinect Inc. and has developed a reputation as an acute observer and interpreter of organizational behaviour in health-care. She applies her knowledge and experience to the development and implementation of learning solutions and assessment tools. These tools support the development of patient-focused cultural change, improved leadership, and team performance. A number of the assessment tools are used in over 200 healthcare organizations across North America.

About the Authors

Index

G

H

I

J

K

L

M

N

O

P

Q

R

U

V

W

X

Z

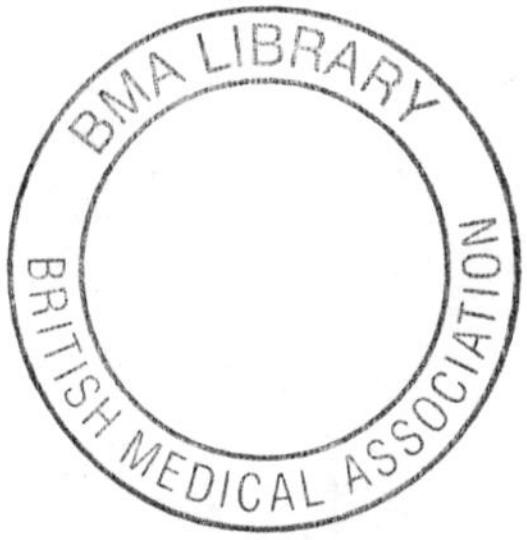